T0249939

"The deep connection with nature's capacity for healing is intrinsic to all life throughout history and across all cultures. In recent times there has been renewed interest from psychotherapists to work with clients in nature. In this exciting new book, arts therapists Ian Siddons Heginworth and Gary Nash have chosen a collection of essays on Environmental Arts Therapy introducing new fresh voices to the discipline. As the practice develops and each Environmental Arts therapist forges a way with diverse emerging perspectives, there is simultaneously a return to older traditions where the wise elders are taking people back into nature for healing and growth. Our flourishing community of Environmental Arts therapists describe and reflect on their various considered and creative approaches."

– Hephzibah Kaplan, *Art Therapist and Director of the London Art Therapy Centre*

"This book is an exciting addition to the growing literature on environmental arts therapies. The editors show how this movement has become an established form of arts therapy, drawing on previous work by others, and leading to their environmental arts therapy course, the first of its kind, based on the cycle of the year. The book also contains fresh voices taking environmental arts therapies into new contexts. At a time of global environmental crisis, this book paves the way to a new way of envisioning therapy, showing the benefits of taking people and therapy out into nature, or bringing nature into the therapy room. It reminds us of the importance of our environment – not an optional extra but the ground of our being."

– Dr Marian Liebmann, OBE, *Art Therapist, teacher and author of art therapy books*

ENVIRONMENTAL ARTS THERAPY

Environmental Arts Therapy: The Wild Frontiers of the Heart describes what happens when we take the creative arts therapies and the people whom we work with out of doors in order to provide safe, structured and accompanied creative therapeutic healing experiences. The theoretical themes are developed along with illustrated examples of clinical practice across a variety of settings and locations.

The work is introduced and co-edited by a pioneer in the field, Ian Siddons Heginworth, who describes the emergence of environmental arts therapy and its growth across the British Isles supported through the training course based in London. The following 12 chapters are written by contributing authors and creative arts therapy practitioners working with children, adults and elders in schools, adult mental health and private practice in Britain and Europe. A central focus of the book is the clinical populations and settings in which clinicians work, and it also describes the health benefits as well as the challenges faced when working out of doors.

This is a book about the emergence of a new creative therapy modality in the British Isles. It shows the value of working with the natural cycles and seasons, using an integrative arts approach including dramatic enactment, role-play, poetry, art-making with natural materials, storytelling, and the use of bodywork through movement, sound, rhythm and the voice, all held and reflected by our encounters with and in nature. It is about our relationship with nature, creativity and therapeutic healing and is written for trainers, trainees and practitioners in the creative arts, psychotherapy and ecotherapy.

Ian Siddons Heginworth is the author of *Environmental Arts Therapy and the Tree of Life*, the book that has inspired the growth of the environmental arts therapy movement in the UK. He leads the postgraduate certificate course in environmental arts therapy at the London Art Therapy Centre and runs a private practice in Devon.

Gary Nash is an art therapist and educator in art and environmental arts therapy training. He co-founded the London Art Therapy Centre in 2009 where he is Clinical Co-Director providing individual art therapy, supervision and group environmental arts therapy.

ENVIRONMENTAL ARTS THERAPY

The Wild Frontiers of the Heart

*Edited by Ian Siddons Heginworth
and Gary Nash*

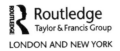

Routledge
Taylor & Francis Group

LONDON AND NEW YORK

First published 2020
by Routledge
2 Park Square, Milton Park, Abingdon, Oxon OX14 4RN

and by Routledge
52 Vanderbilt Avenue, New York, NY 10017

Routledge is an imprint of the Taylor & Francis Group, an informa business

© 2020 selection and editorial matter, Ian Siddons Heginworth and
Gary Nash; individual chapters, the contributors

The right of Ian Siddons Heginworth and Gary Nash; to be identified as
the authors of the editorial material, and of the authors for their individual
chapters, has been asserted in accordance with sections 77 and 78 of the
Copyright, Designs and Patents Act 1988.

All rights reserved. No part of this book may be reprinted or reproduced or
utilised in any form or by any electronic, mechanical, or other means, now
known or hereafter invented, including photocopying and recording, or in
any information storage or retrieval system, without permission in writing
from the publishers.

Trademark notice: Product or corporate names may be trademarks or
registered trademarks, and are used only for identification and explanation
without intent to infringe.

British Library Cataloguing-in-Publication Data
A catalogue record for this book is available from the British Library

Library of Congress Cataloging-in-Publication Data
A catalog record for this book has been requested

ISBN: 978-1-138-34584-3 (hbk)
ISBN: 978-1-138-34586-7 (pbk)
ISBN: 978-0-429-43764-9 (ebk)

Typeset in Bembo
by Apex CoVantage, LLC

Cover image entitled 'Spears' photo taken by
Gary Nash, 2016

CONTENTS

List of illustrations   x
Contributors   xi
Foreword by Mary-Jayne Rust   xv
Acknowledgements   xx

   Introduction by the editors   1
   Ian Siddons Heginworth and Gary Nash

PART I
Environmental arts therapy in context   **7**

1 Turning: the emergence and growth of environmental
   arts therapy in the British Isles   9
   Ian Siddons Heginworth

2 Weaving the threads of theory and experience: a review
   of the literature   27
   Gary Nash

PART II
Childhood, love and attachment: the heart of the matter 45

3 The wild inside: offering children natural materials and an ecopsychological understanding of self within art therapy 47
Lydia Boon

4 EarthWays: environmental arts therapy for repairing insecure attachment and developing creative response-ability in an insecure world 61
Lia Ponton

5 Bringing the outside in: reflecting upon Mother within a pilot group in environmental arts therapy 79
Michelle Edinburgh

PART III
Feminine and masculine: putting feeling first 91

6 Meeting the wounded feminine: trauma-informed environmental arts therapy as an approach to working with physical illness 93
Susie Thompson

7 The wood between the worlds: encountering the wounded healer in environmental arts therapy 106
William Secretan

8 The tapping on the window: environmental arts therapy and the integrated self 121
Auriel Eagleton

PART IV
The cycle of the year: working with the seasons 135

9 Taking art therapy outdoors: a Circle of Trees 137
Gary Nash

10 Creating connections: introducing environmental
    arts therapy into London's green spaces   151
    Simon Woodward

11 Space to move, explore and create: taking art therapy into
    the outdoor environment in adult mental health services   167
    Pamela Stanley

PART V
Elders and endings: the wild road on   **183**

12 Trees of life and death: a journey into the heart of
    Transylvania to use environmental arts therapy
    with groups of adults and staff in palliative care   185
    Hannah Monteiro

13 Growing elders: the cultivation and collaboration
    of an elder women's group in the woods   197
    Deborah Kelly and Vanessa Jones

    Epilogue   214
    Ian Siddons Heginworth

Index   *217*

ILLUSTRATIONS

Table

8.1   Contact styles   129

Figures

1.1   Child in matchbox   13
1.2   Spears   16
1.3   Reed boat   24
3.1   Nature mask   51
4.1   Magic imp   75
5.1   Tree with skulls   84
5.2   Weed   85
9.1   Natural materials in the opening circle   141
9.2   Land art, leaf, soil and sticks   144
9.3   Natural artwork assembled indoors   147
10.1   Luke's artwork   156
10.2   Chloe's artwork   157
10.3   Leah's artwork   165
11.1   Heartfelt, a body map experience in response to December's descent in 2016   168
12.1   A weary tree   190
12.2   Forest   191
12.3   Nurture   194
12.4   Leaf of death   195
13.1   Staffs   202
13.2   Woman walking in woods   204

CONTRIBUTORS

Lydia Boon is a registered art psychotherapist working with children and adolescents in schools. She completed her initial degree in creative expressive therapies in 2007, having focussed her research on a synthesis of ecopsychological and creative expressive therapy. She completed her art psychotherapy MA in 2014, which included research into the use of clay in art psychotherapy for those having experienced early relational trauma, and subsequently went on to complete the training in environmental arts therapy at the London Art Therapy Centre. Lydia is currently developing her practice running therapy groups outdoors. A deep familiarity with her own art practice, extensive experience providing group and 1:1 therapy, combining elements of art, creative expression and engagement with outer and inner nature continues to enrich her therapeutic approach.

Auriel Eagleton, MAIAP, is a HCPC registered integrative arts psychotherapist. She uses a combination of art forms including dance, movement, drama, music, creative writing, clay work, painting and sandplay to facilitate self-expression in her practice. She subsequently trained in environmental arts therapy and extended her practice outdoors. Auriel uses a Buddhist orientation to support her understanding of the ways in which people can grow and heal through awareness of and contact with Nature. She works with both adults and children and has a special interest in the ways in which physical movement through painting, and in contact with the elements in outdoor settings, can facilitate well-being and support the therapeutic process. Auriel is a co-founder of The Woodland Retreat in London, a sustainable arts studio set in Queens Woods, North London, providing a space for pioneering nature-based therapies to be practised in the city.

Michelle Edinburgh, MAAP, is a HCPC registered art psychotherapist and environmental art therapy practitioner who is employed in adult mental health services in Plymouth, Devon. She also works in private practice from a workshop in her garden on the edge of the city and runs monthly women's eco art therapy groups in Dartmoor National Park. She loves to sing, dance, paint and create. She walks the land as much as possible and seeks to bring the wild both literally and metaphorically into her practice as much as possible.

Ian Siddons Heginworth, RDTh, MPhil, is an environmental arts therapist and storyteller. He is the author of *Environmental Arts Therapy and the Tree of Life*, the book that has become the flagship of the environmental arts therapy movement in the UK, and *Hairy Tales*, a collection of original fairy stories. In 2016 after 35 years he retired from the National Health Service (NHS) where he had been employed as a specialist practitioner developing outdoor therapeutic services for adults with profound and complex disabilities, and for adults with enduring mental health issues, in wild and beautiful locations all over Devon. He now leads the postgraduate certificate course in environmental arts therapy at the London Art Therapy Centre and runs a private practice as an environmental arts therapist in therapeutic woodland near Exeter.

Vanessa Jones, Dip AT, MAAT, is a HCPC registered art therapist with over 20 years clinical experience. She has developed several long-standing outdoor art therapy groups for adults within NHS mental health services, building a body of evidence from these concurrent projects over eight years. She facilitates workshops and trainings in London and holds a monthly environmental arts therapy practice group in North London. Vanessa is published in professional literature and is currently completing a masters study into art, nature and grief.

Deborah Kelly is a UKCP integrative arts psychotherapist, teacher and supervisor. Deborah has worked in and with nature and the imagination for the past 20 years, running numerous bereavement, shiatsu and women's groups. She established and facilitates two palliative care projects, working with nature, myth and the rhythm of the seasons. This work, with particular emphasis on the nature of therapeutic space, has been the subject of her doctoral research and published writing. Deborah runs a private practice in East Sussex and teaches in London.

Hannah Monteiro is a HCPC registered art psychotherapist who trained at the University of Derby, qualifying in 2014. Her background is working in forensic, palliative, educational and charity settings with children, young people and adults who have experienced complex trauma and bereavement. She has adopted a psychodynamic, psychoanalytic approach intertwined with narrative, myth and metaphor. In addition to her art psychotherapy practice, Hannah facilitates psycho-educational, self-care and creative art-making workshops for clients, students and staff groups. In 2018, she was invited back as a visiting lecturer to the University of Derby to facilitate an outdoor art-making and reflective workshop as part of the MA art therapy program. Hannah has a special interest in cross-cultural work, bringing art therapy outdoors and exploring the magical metaphors that grow from natural materials.

Gary Nash Dip AT, MAAT, is a HCPC registered art therapist, supervisor and private practitioner. He trained in 1989 and 1995 at Goldsmiths and St Albans. He has developed a private practice since 1995 alongside his work in social services, the voluntary sector and mainstream education. Gary co-founded the London Art Therapy Centre in 2009 where he is clinical co-director providing individual and group art therapy and delivering professional workshops and training for arts therapists. He has developed an integrated arts therapy practice which uses methods and approaches derived from the environmental arts therapy training that he completed in 2014.

Lia Ponton is a HCPC registered dramatherapist and environmental arts therapist. Including her private practice, Lia works with children in care and education and young adults with learning disabilities. Lia has an environmental arts therapy practice in the Devon countryside. She also has experience combining the arts therapies with equine therapy. Lia has had links with environmental activism from a young age and is a member of the local Inner Transition Core group, supporting the community by exploring inner psychological and emotional responses to outer crises (climate change, peak oil, war) and examining how inner processes shape and influence the outer transition to making our systems for transport, food, energy and shelter more sustainable and healthier. She is also a qualified playback theatre practitioner working in diverse communities, including refugees and women who have experienced domestic violence. She lives on a farm on Dartmoor.

William Secretan, MA, is a HCPC registered dramatherapist and works in the NHS as an arts psychotherapist within a specialist psychology and psychological therapies service. He works with adults experiencing severe, complex and enduring mental distress. William originally trained in wilderness therapy, from 2003–2005, before later training in dramatherapy, environmental arts therapy and psychodrama psychotherapy. He has worked for several years with both groups and individuals, exploring the healing aspects of myth-enactment and ritual in outdoor settings. William has lived off-grid and worked in many outdoor settings in the UK, Australia and New Zealand. He has been an environmental activist and is a lifelong student of British folklore and customs.

Pamela Stanley, MAAP, is a HCPC registered art psychotherapist and environmental arts therapist living and working in Snowdonia, North Wales. She has been employed by the NHS in adult mental health for 16 years working with in-patients and in the community to establish a meaningful practice as part of a broader arts therapy service and has developed art therapy groups in collaboration with community services and local authorities. She trained to move her art therapy practice outdoors into the natural environment with the aim to creating and developing a dynamic group process actively working with all the senses, the mind and the body. Having recently retired from the NHS she continues to work as a sessional practitioner with Nature providing a creative and restorative space.

Susie Thompson is a HCPC registered dramatherapist, trainer and coach working in private practice with individuals, groups and organisations. She works with adults and young people supporting those with life challenges; physical illnesses, including chronic fatigue syndrome/myalgic encephalomyelitis; mental health difficulties; and learning disabilities. Her special interest is in trauma (and chronic stress), and she has developed a creative mind-body approach. Susie runs women's circles, groups and workshops in shamanic journeying and ritual, and environmental arts therapy as well as group dramatherapy for adults with learning disabilities and for young people combining dramatherapy and equine therapy (equi-dramatherapy). She works in south Devon where she lives with her husband and son and in Leicestershire on the land that raised her. She is passionate about helping people to connect with stories and the natural world to enable them to access their wild and wise selves.

Simon Woodward, MA, is a HCPC registered art psychotherapist and British Association of Art Therapists BAAT accredited private practitioner. He is a co-founder of the Community Outdoor Art Therapy Service (COATS), which has provided nature-based well-being groups, facilitated workshops for therapists looking to take their practice outdoors, run seasonal outdoor workshops and provided therapeutic art-making workshops in London for both adults and children. He supervises MA art therapy trainees in a university setting as well as facilitating Jungian workshops and delivering lectures on outdoor art therapy. His current professional practice includes facilitating group outdoor art therapy on a college farm for students who have additional educational needs. Simon also provides private individual outdoor and indoor art therapy.

FOREWORD

Forests are living communities of magnificent beings. Each giant being has its own character, its own texture of bark, its own pattern of leaves and colour of green creating carpets of red-orange-brown in their fall. Forests provide food, shelter, wisdom and sanctuary for all kinds of life including humans. Recent scientific research confirms ancient knowledge that in any forest the trees are in communication with each other via the 'Wood Wide Web' (McFarlane, 2016).

Perhaps trees can communicate with humans too, if we know how to listen. Clarissa Pinkola Estes describes how:

> In the old country, where my parents came from, my father said the big trees were "Guardian Trees". All villages had Guardian Trees at the beginning of the road leading to the little houses. The sound of the wind in the leaves of the trees or the needles in the evergreens would change if people were coming from a distance, walking or on wagon or on horseback. The Guardian Trees would tell when someone was far off but advancing toward the village, and from which direction, and on what kind of conveyance, and sometimes whether they were armed or not.
>
> (Pinkola Estes, 2010)

Listening to the more-than-human world means listening with our senses. When I cross from urban tarmac into forest, the air is filled with bird conversations and the rustling of trees; the smell of leaves permeates my nostrils, and in every step my senses are awakened. What petty concerns might have been occupying my mind begin to drift away as I sink more deeply into my body. I am, for the time being, transformed. As the trees and I exchange our breath, I begin to see that there is no sharp dividing line between my skin-encapsulated 'self' and the rest of nature. The small 'I' is now in relation to the larger self; things have come back into perspective.

"Dod yn ôl at fy nghoed" is a Welsh phrase which means "to return to a balanced state of mind", but literally means "to return to my trees".

The forest offers many teachings: the art of being deeply rooted in place, or the art of shedding skin and drawing in energy for winter, or a different perspective on time. Slowing down enables the art of noticing, such as the wonder of synchronous connections: a queen wasp arrives just when my client is lost for words in telling me about her stinging mother. Everyone within the forest community has something to say: squirrels, birds, insects, dogs walking their humans, as well as the infinite blue of sky. This is a place where the soul can be spoken to and re-charged, where the rational mind can let go and allow a more playful spirit in. This is not a 'cure-all' but more an offering to the imagination, a way of finding meaning in our world too full of suffering.

The woods can also bring a sense of darkness and foreboding: from Mirkwood in *The Lord of the Rings* to *Little Red Riding Hood*, such stories remind us that the forest offers a place of adventure where humans meet their shadow selves.

What better place in which to practice therapy?

It is therefore with great pleasure that I am writing the foreword to this anthology about environmental arts therapy. Forests have been its birthplace, and the variety of writings here show that environmental arts therapy is spreading to other habitats too, as well as benefitting many different kinds of clients and therapeutic work.

This new development in the profession of arts therapies comes not a moment too soon. What you will find in this book (pages courtesy of trees) are descriptions of the countless ways in which environmental arts therapy offers healing in the midst of The Great Climate Crisis: it fosters imagination, metaphorical thinking, story-telling, embodiment, creativity and play as well as a chance to return to a deeper relationship with the more-than-human world, all vital for our troubled souls in troubled times.

Playing in the woods or on the beach, making art with found objects, allows our whole body-mind to relax and to free associate. This is the place of new insights, dreams and radical new ideas. Jung writes:

> At any time in my later life when I came up against a blank wall, I painted a picture or hewed stone. Each such experience proved to be a rite d'entrée for the ideas and work that followed hard upon it. Everything that I have written this year and last year . . . has grown out of the stone sculptures I did after my wife's death. The close of her life . . . wrenched me violently out of myself. It cost me a great deal to regain my footing and contact with stone helped me.
> *(Jung, 1967, pp. 198–199)*

Yet from the moment children are sent to school they are taught that indoors is the place for 'real' work and outdoors is for play. This lays the foundation for a toxic split between rational, focused, linear thought located in the mind and a more diffuse, creative consciousness which emerges from the body-mind. Gradually we are taught that it is rational thinking that really matters in life while play, imagination and creativity is what happens in the gaps between real work. Sadly, even these gaps in which we have always been free to dream are now being filled with mobile phone fiddling.

So it is vitally important that we remember the awe, wonder, mystery and wisdom that the other-than-human world inspires; sitting at the foot of a tree, for example, looking up and watching its canopy swaying in the breeze – this simple experience can shift a stuck inner state enough to loosen and work with it. In times of grief, anger, depression or anxiety, sitting in the garden or in a local park can enable a shift in perspective. My client, who was in the midst of mourning the loss of her partner, could see no new life ahead. In that moment an acorn dropped into her lap. These moments of simplicity can speak more than a thousand words.

Environmental arts therapy, along with other forms of ecotherapy, naturally invites us to re-vision the notion of the self as ecological: we are interconnected and interdependent with the rest of nature from the moment we are conceived in our mothers' watery wombs. For too long we have been under the spell that we are separate from, and superior to, the other-than-human world. This story of separation is deeply embedded within our mind-set and our language, revealed, for example, when we talk about 'going out into nature'. Yet we only need to hold our breath for longer than a few minutes to know that we are in nature, and part of nature, all the time.

How can we find language to heal our dualistic ways of seeing? Just as the past 100 years of psychotherapy has created a language to describe the multitude of inner-world states and interpersonal dynamics, so the diverse range of ecotherapies are starting to create new languages for our relationship with 'nature'. This anthology is part of building this new way of seeing.

For example, we have this one word 'nature' which has many different meanings: the natural world as opposed to the human-made world; our intrinsic human nature or essence. The root of the word nature is *natus* meaning birth; nature is the birthplace of our species, and it is the place to which we return at the end of life. Indigenous peoples remind us that nature is not just a physical body but sacred also, often signified by using a capital N. Nature means the greater whole in which we live, the Great Mystery. Here, too, I am fumbling for words to describe the ineffable, the divine, none of them quite fitting. We need more nuanced words to match our experience and imaginations.

Another key part of environmental arts therapy is facing the shadow. Entering my local urban forest, the litter is just one manifestation of the shadow of consumer culture, a reminder of the schisms between humans and the rest of nature, the lack of care for the Earth. One day, my client Rachel assembled a range of plastic items found on the forest floor. She broke down and wept as she told me,

> There is no wild place left on the planet that is untouched by human greed and lack of care. I try my best to care but everything I use and buy is part of this destructive system and it's just getting worse. I can't bear it anymore. Sometimes I think it would be much better if humans were just wiped out.

As we sat together under the strength of the oak exploring more of Rachel's despair, grief and anger, a blackbird perched on a black plastic bag amidst her artwork and sang with the clearest of notes. In this poignant moment Rachel realised that beauty and destructiveness are intrinsic to everything and everyone in nature, including humans, including herself. This recognition allowed her to move out of a place of wanting all humans to be gone and into a place of wanting to defend the web of life in which we have our rightful place. Eventually she found her niche in taking creative action; there she found a different kind of hope which is more about living in the present and in relationship.

Our shadow is also evident in how easy it is to take the earth for granted, like an adolescent in relation to mother. For this reason, I invite my clients to stand with me at the threshold of the woods at the start of every session. We ask the trees (out loud or silently) if we can enter, if they will support us in our therapeutic journey, or whatever words seem right at the time. At the end of the session we thank the forest. This might be surprising for some, but it is a reminder that we are entering into a relationship rather than a place which could be seen as a 'set of tools' or 'resources' for the inner work of therapy subsumed into another kind of consumerism.

Along similar lines, nature writer Richard Mabey cautions against a simplistic version of ecotherapy which suggests that all we have to do is go out on a sunny day and look at the pretty bluebell wood and everything will be OK. He continues,

> This is not only insulting to the complexity of human beings but also deeply insulting to the complexity of nature ... This spring has been devastating for wildlife. ... the young will be dying of cold and exposure in the nests ... if we are willing to realise that the natural world, too, has its moments of profound recession then I think this does bring with it a kind of psychological maturation about what it means to be a living thing which is surely the most profound psychological lesson anyone can learn.
>
> *(Mabey, 2012)*

I hope this anthology illustrates the many layers of this complexity to the reader.

Just as one of the tasks of psychotherapy might be to help a client come home to themselves, perhaps one of the many tasks of ecotherapy is to explore and come home to nature, to help individuals find their place again in the great scheme of things. It also helps us come to know ourselves as animals, and to come to love and respect our animal nature as well as respecting the wisdom of the more-than-human world. We do this by realising we are part of the great round of seasons, of life and death. There is no greater teacher than this.

by Mary-Jayne Rust April 2019

Mary-Jayne Rust is an ecopsychologist and psychotherapist inspired by trainings in art therapy, feminist psychotherapy and Jungian analysis. Journeys to Ladakh (on the Tibetan plateau) in the early 1990s alerted her to the seriousness of the ecological crisis and its cultural, economic and spiritual roots. Alongside her therapy practice she runs courses and lectures internationally on ecopsychology, a growing field of inquiry into the psychological dimensions of ecological crisis. Her publications can be found on www.mjrust.net, including *Vital Signs: Psychological Responses to Ecological Crisis* (Rust and Totton, 2012).

She grew up beside the sea and is wild about swimming. Now she lives and works beside ancient woodland in North London.

References

Jung, C.G. (1967). *Memories, dreams, reflections*. London & Glasgow: Fontana Library of Theology and Philosophy.

Mabey, R. (2012). Interview 'Not all in the mind'. *BBC Sounds*. Retrieved 17 March 2019, from: www.bbc.co.uk/programmes/b01k1nl3.

McFarlane, R. (2016). The secrets of the wood wide web. *The New Yorker* (7 August, 2016).

Pinkola Estes, C. (2010). Insights at the edge podcast. Interview with Tami Simon, Sounds True.

Rust, M.J., and Totton, N. (2012). *Vital signs: Psychological responses to ecological crisis*. London: Karnac Books.

ACKNOWLEDGEMENTS

We would like to share our appreciation of the many people who have supported the growth and emergence of this work and this book. We would firstly like to thank Mary-Jayne Rust for writing the foreword, Hephzibah Kaplan and her colleagues at the London Art Therapy Centre for their continuing support over many years whilst developing and providing the training programme, and Jonathan Meares and his team at Highgate Wood for allowing us to set up our tent tepee and work among the trees. We would also like to thank everyone who has contributed to the course either by leading workshops or by giving feedback to student essays, including Vanessa Jones and Simon Woodward. Thanks are also due to Simon for bravely grappling with the more complex technical editing tasks.

In no way does this book represent the totality of environmental arts therapy practice here in the British Isles and we would like to honour all the practitioners out there who, having completed the London course, are now developing their practice in the wild frontiers of the heart, pushing back the boundaries of what it means to be human in relation to nature. This is deep adaptation on the front line, at a time when we are needing it most, and we are profoundly grateful to you all.

I (Ian) remain deeply indebted to Gary for his inspired holding of the London course, without which I would probably still be soldiering away by myself in the woods. As ever I wish to thank and truly honour the lion-hearted souls who come to work with me there among the shadows, and also the other-than-human co-therapists, some clad in fur, some in feather, some in leaves and some in slime, shine or shimmer, who dip in and out of our sessions as therapeutic synchronicity requires. I would also like to thank Devon Partnership Trust, who did exactly that, trusting me to develop a completely new and experimental practice whilst under their wings.

I (Gary) wish to share my appreciation of my working partnership with Ian who continues to inspire my practice through his words and actions. My heartfelt gratitude goes out to Martin Jordan for his commitment to making his work accessible to a wider audience and to Shaun McNiff for showing how we complete the creative-nature-healing cycle for me personally.

We would both like to thank our wives/partners and children for their enduring patience and support while we were lost to them in this Herculean labour, and also our colleagues, clients and communities for their continued encouragement. Finally, we wish to acknowledge Nature, with a capital N, who stands beside, around and within us always, guiding and teaching us constantly, and who has, we suspect, her own agenda in this matter, and of course the indigenous peoples of the world who have been doing this kind of thing forever.

INTRODUCTION BY THE EDITORS

Ian Siddons Heginworth and Gary Nash

Environmental arts therapy is an arts-based approach to working therapeutically in outdoor spaces and emerges from the creative exchange that has occurred between the ecopsychology movement and the arts therapies professions and communities. This book represents the gentle and committed tending of an approach to working therapeutically in, with and through nature developed over several decades. Although the term is relatively new, environmental arts therapy draws deeply from an ancient history, a timeframe in which human experience has always sought expression through different art forms in relationship with the natural world. At the heart of this approach is an acknowledgement of the complexity of human psychology and a recognition of the 'wildness' found in human nature.

When we step outside of our studios and consulting rooms we find, as the chapters in this book will describe, that our approaches, methods and sensitivities are shaped by the dynamic forces of nature. These forces can be subtle and gentle or sudden and dramatic. The changeable qualities are ever present and on one hand this provides both therapist and client with a profound emotional and sensory experience of the unpredictable; of change, uncertainty and transition. This in itself is a great teaching. But the real power and mystery of this work lies in the synchronistic resonance between what is emerging inwardly in the feeling self at any given time and what we then encounter before us or unfolding around us in nature. Clients are naturally drawn to the locations that best reflect their inner struggle and invariably find there the materials and natural encounters that best allow the work to unfold. They find too in the natural metaphors offered by the turning of the year and the mythologies that accompany it, a deeper meaning for their own emotional process. It is through this dialogue, where the inner world is met, made and interacted with outwardly that the deep transformational work of environmental arts therapy is made manifest.

Environmental arts therapy is by its very nature an integrative creative arts therapy, one where we use all of the arts to further therapeutic intention. Through the act of moving outdoors we experience all of our senses. As the work of therapy deepens it is facilitated through a focused attention and gentle attunement to what we find and how it resonates with feeling, affect and imagination. The healing processes inherent in this experience are mobilised through the senses and developed further as we offer those we work with an invitation to respond through the arts. Creative expression may involve dramatic enactment, role-play, sculpting or art-making with natural materials, storytelling, and the use of bodywork through movement, sound, rhythm and the voice, all held and reflected by what we find in nature.

The therapeutic combination of the arts and nature, human and other-than-human, is informed by a growing awareness and interest in the work of ecopsychology which considers our interdependency and interrelationship with the Earth. The philosophy underpinning this approach is driven by bigger questions around human consciousness and relationships beyond the self, a necessary development within psychotherapy as the balance between human activity and life sustaining ecologies are threatened. Theodor Roszak raises questions regarding the limits of conventional psychotherapy, psychology and counselling and challenges us to consider widening our perspective:

> For psychologists and therapists, their understanding of human sanity has always stopped at the city limits. The creation of an urban intellect and intending to heal urban angst, modern psychotherapy has never seen fit to reach beyond family and society to address the non-human habitat that so engulfs the tiny psychic island.
>
> *(Roszak, 1995, p. 2)*

As we open the studio door and step outside, we seek to shift the restrictions inherent in the conventional clinical paradigm, a paradigm within which clients come to receive and therapists are employed to give. Instead, with nature as co therapist, we collaboratively seek a greater sense of knowing, sharing and healing together. When we add ritual, mythology, imagination and art to the relational work of psychotherapy outdoors, alongside an understanding of the turning wheel of the year, we generate another intrinsically healing cycle of energy. We find ourselves consistently reflected in all that we make, encounter or find, and through sharing and being witnessed in our creativity we ritualise and manifest change. Creativity, like nature herself, provides stimulus and frustration as we, both as clients and therapists, confront the despair and beauty pulsing through the human heart.

Environmental Arts Therapy: The Wild Frontiers of the Heart has been written and edited by creative arts therapists who have a primary training in either drama or art therapy. Nearly all have also had further training in environmental arts therapy. All authors are registered and practising therapists working in different settings and contexts. Each practitioner has developed their own approach to taking their creative arts practice out of doors and have shaped their practice according to the needs of their client group, their particular clinical interests and by the restraints provided by the settings and environments in which they work.

In Chapter 1 the individual therapy work described takes place in private therapeutic woodland with adults in Devon. The author tells the story of how his own practice developed, both within the National Health Service (NHS) with adult mental health service users and in private practice, marking the beginnings of environmental arts therapy in the British Isles, and how through the training course this approach is now growing throughout the country.

The literature review in Chapter 2 provides a theoretical context for the work and the approaches used considering also the challenges faced when taking clinical practice outdoors, the health benefits and evidence-base. There are important questions around efficacy, risk and professional boundaries alongside practitioners' views as to how we respond creatively and ethically when we radically alter the therapeutic frame.

Chapter 3 describes three case studies, supported by research in child development, to explore the ways in which bringing a selection of natural materials into the art therapy room and incorporating ecopsychological concepts of self adds something new, vital and important to art therapy with children.

In Chapter 4 the themes of play and ritual are explored in relation to attachment patterns and developmental trauma through a wider relational context when working outdoors, considering also the part that this can play in developing a personal response to climate trauma.

Chapter 5 discusses an eighteen-week environmental arts therapy pilot group with adult mental health clients, using both traditional art materials and nature as its primary mode of relating. A central theme which emerges is in relation to mother, the impact of hostile mothering and the group's tentative connections to the Earth as great mother.

Chapter 6 considers the potential for trauma-informed environmental arts therapy to help reduce the pain and symptoms of clients suffering with chronic fatigue syndrome/myalgic encephalomyelitis (CFS/ME), highlighting research that shows how childhood trauma and emotional suppression contribute to these conditions. It tells the story of what happens during a single case study involving ten sessions, describing the resulting significant improvements made to the symptoms and physical energy levels of the participating client.

The author in Chapter 7 examines his own experience of being a client in one-to-one environmental arts therapy working within a frame of 'men's work': using body, power and positive risk-taking. It presents a therapeutic exploration of childhood trauma, domestic violence and parental suicide and demonstrates how environmental arts therapy can be used as a profound and effective method of exploration and change.

The 'Circle of Trees' model described in Chapter 1 is developed in the next four chapters. The use of storytelling to bridge the inner world and the world around us, whilst working with the cycle of the seasons, provides a central theme to Chapter 8.

The feminine and masculine principles, here defined as solar and lunar time, are described in the context of working outdoors.

The cycle of the seasons and the deepening of one's attunement with the transitions and changes which are naturally occurring provide the structure for Chapter 9. Working with the themes provided by the trees and cultural stories associated with them, therapeutic work with adults and the training of environmental arts therapists is described.

Chapter 10 describes how the author set up COATS, the Community Outdoor Art Therapy Service in London, using urban parks and community gardens. Working with the British seasonal changes and the different projects, their themes and exercises are described, while reflecting on the health benefits available to us when working out of doors.

Chapter 11 is also focused on adult mental health services. This chapter provides an insight into the key stages and methodologies that have supported the development of an established environmental arts therapy practice within the Art Therapies Service in Adult Mental Health, Betsi Cadwaladr University Health Board, North Wales.

The final two chapters move towards the end of the life cycle, Chapter 12 is based in Romania in a hospice setting with terminally ill adult patients and the staff who care for them. It gives an account of using natural materials and 'The Tree of Life' model for patient and staff support groups, enabling them to share their feelings and begin to talk about death. The individual trees then become united in a forest of personal stories.

Chapter 13 explores the development of an elder women's group working in and with woodland to explore and celebrate womanhood and aging. It is written from the perspective of its facilitators including voices of group participants. The chapter explores how the group process and facilitation style unfolded into a collaborative and co-created space for ritual, creativity and community.

Environmental Arts Therapy: The Wild Frontiers of the Heart is a book about the emergence of a new creative therapy modality in the British Isles. But wherever we are on this beautiful yet ailing Earth, on whatever landmass or continent and in whichever hemisphere, there will always be twelve months in the year and thirteen lunar cycles; there will always be beginnings and endings, the turning of the seasons marked by the gradual movement of the Earth around the sun. When we attune to these we find that nature has something to share with us. Wherever we are situated we will find that human cultural narratives have emerged and evolved in relation to these cycles and still speak to us about the deep and enduring relationship between our inner and outer worlds. When we remember this we find ourselves held and in context, not only in natural space, but in natural time as well.

When we attune to nature and the cultural narratives which reflect the natural cycles of life within and around us, we re-attune to the possibility of a reciprocal reconnection with the Earth, enhancing our human and other-than-human relationships. The simplicity of this relational ecology is described succinctly by Shaun McNiff: "As we give respect and attention to our physical and natural environments, there is a corresponding effect on our selves" (McNiff, 2017, p. iv). This reciprocal cycle of energy between self, other and other-than-human is at the heart of environmental arts therapy and reflects the work described and the experiences shared by each author on the pages of this book.

As the science relating to climate change makes ever grimmer reading (Bendell, 2018), there has never been a more important time to cultivate this. As we struggle to reconcile our role in, and responsibility for, the current environmental crisis both we and the natural world yearn for the opportunity to heal together. This book, and the practice that it describes, has grown from that yearning.

References

Bendell, J. (2018). *Deep adaptation: A map for navigating climate change.* IFLAS occasional paper 2. Retrieved from: www.IFLAS.info.

McNiff, S. (2017). Foreword. In Kopytin, A., and Rugh, M. (Eds.), *Environmental expressive therapies: Nature assisted theory and practice.* New York and Oxon: Routledge.

Roszak, T. (1995). Where psyche meets Gaia. In Roszak, T., Gomes, M., and Kanner, A.D. (Eds.), *Ecopsychology: Restoring the earth, healing the mind* (pp. 1–17). San Francisco, CA: Sierra Club Books.

PART I

Environmental arts therapy in context

1

TURNING

The emergence and growth of environmental arts therapy in the British Isles

Ian Siddons Heginworth

Introduction

Given the opportunity every child will play in the mud, the sand and the snow. Leaf mounds, sand castles, dams in the stream, dens in the wood and fairy houses in the trees; these are so often our primary experiences of making and shaping in the world around us, the means by which we first express our inner world outwardly. This will be true in one form or other throughout the world and throughout both the history and prehistory of humanity. Environmental art is our indigenous art form and when we return to it we return to something vital and primal within ourselves. In over twenty years of practice the phrase that I have most often heard repeated by clients rediscovering this art form is 'it feels like coming home'.

I am an environmental art therapist with a private practice in Devon, England. Environmental arts therapy is an arts-based ecotherapy which has grown from the roots of the ecopsychology movement. The first published use of the term 'environmental arts therapy' was in the article Environmental Arts Therapy, Metaphors in the Field, by Jean Davies (1999). In 2008 I published *Environmental Arts Therapy and the Tree of Life*, a book about my own practice which is aligned wholly to the turning of the year (the cycle of the seasons) and this has led to the emergence and growth of environmental arts therapy as a new therapeutic modality here in the British Isles. This introduction tells that story.

In this chapter I will gently trace the cycle of the turning year here in the British Isles and touch lightly on some of the natural metaphors traditionally associated with each month (metaphors inspired by the unfolding of natural processes as the year turns), naming some of the traditional festivals related to this cycle. On the postgraduate certificate in environmental arts therapy course that takes place in London, we explore many such metaphors drawn from the Celtic and other traditions that once accompanied this turning and so serve still as an indigenous frame of reference for these northern European forests. In my environmental arts therapy practice I only occasionally use my understanding of these metaphors (unless I am teaching them) to direct the therapeutic process, for this must always come from the authentic experience of the client, but there can be great healing in reflecting on them at the end of the session, where people can begin to see that feelings or behaviour that they had deemed to be dysfunctional and problematic are aligned to a greater cycle. Also, I always aim to move towards the release and expression of feeling and, when this is well hidden, the appearance in someone's work of a metaphor relevant to the time of year is usually a fair indicator of where it might be found.

Interspersed with this will be anecdotes and vignettes from my own experience as an environmental arts therapist, trainer and client to illustrate the unique nature of the practice, with a particular emphasis on relationship with the inner child and the therapeutic release of anger, the latter an area in which, in my opinion, environmental arts therapy excels, for nature is the primary safe container for wildness. The vignettes come with the permission of those involved, but have been heavily disguised to ensure confidentiality. Running alongside all will be a further narrative telling the story of my own practice and the subsequent growth of environmental arts therapy here in the British Isles. Finally, I will reflect upon the role that environmental arts therapy has to play in responding to the environmental crisis. As the ecosystems that sustain us and all life on Earth begin to fail under the strain that we place upon them, can there be a more important time to marry our healing with that of the planet, using the metaphorical and transformative language of the arts to realign our inner nature with our outer? In our increasingly secular and technologically driven world the fusion of art, nature and therapy welcomes ritual, mystery and meaning back into our lives, helping us to reconnect to the natural world, to natural cycles and consequently, to our natural selves.

In environmental arts therapy 'turning' is at the heart of all, as it is for each of us throughout our lives from beginning to end. At the moment of human conception, when the sperm fertilizes the ovum, something extraordinary and mysterious happens (Avinoam, 2002). The egg begins to turn upon its axis like the Earth spinning in space. It is as if the first fusion of masculine and feminine, the re-cementing of the duality of life into a single unity once again begins the turning that is inherent in all things, a turning that defines life itself. As if turning and living are synonymous. After all, the universe turns, indeed the word universe means 'the Turning One'. We turn when we begin and we are turning now, not just within the boundless sweep of the stars, not just upon this spinning Earth, but around the sun as well. In consequence the seasons turn around and within us, compelling our feeling selves to follow and explore, quite independently of our intent, the varied shades and textures of our humanity. And the moon, she circles us all, drawing us into her turning. So it is from the moment of conception to the moment of death we dance like Shiva in his circle of flame.

It is this awareness of the turning cycles of nature and our deep and inherent feeling connection to them that informs and defines environmental arts therapy and makes it so much more than just art therapy outdoors. In the handbook that accompanies the course we write:

> We believe that Environmental Arts Therapy is a new and unique arts therapy that does not fit into any of the existing modalities. This is because: Environmental arts therapy is practiced outdoors (or natural materials and an awareness of natural cycles are brought indoors) and it enjoys a profound and intimate relationship with the natural world, inspired and shaped by the locations that it inhabits. The foundation of environmental arts therapy is its unique relationship with the turning year (the cycle of the seasons) and metaphors, myths and traditions relating to each month, so its therapeutic processes are embedded in the natural passage of time. Environmental arts therapy is multimedia combining: visual arts, drama, movement, voice-work and ritual, all practiced outdoors.
>
> *(Siddons Heginworth et al., 2013, p. 2)*

Composting

Environmental Arts Therapy and the Tree of Life used poetic metaphor to describe the turning year here in these Northern European temperate lands:

> As the days grow short the shadows creep in. The blanket of leaves grows dark and lies like a shroud upon the cold body of the earth as she draws back her fluids into herself. Winter sucks the life out of the land with a harsh and oppressive hunger, and all that is soft and warm recoils in the face of her advance. The woodland creatures hibernate, sealing up their dens to salvage and sustain the heat in themselves. They wrap themselves around it and sleep, little pockets of hot life embedded in the cold clay. Secret dreamers among the black roots, spirits of fur and claw and snuffling snout, cave dwellers, fire keepers, as silent as grubs they hide from winter's fierce and probing tongue.
>
> *(Siddons Heginworth, 2008, p. 30)*

Now we, another seventeen secret dreamers among the black roots, huddle up together to keep warm in our tepee nestled among the trees of a wintry Highgate Wood in London. It is a weekend workshop on the postgraduate certificate in environmental arts therapy course, hosted by the London Art Therapy Centre. This intake of the course is newly started but everyone is dreaming. One by one each participant outlines his or her plans to move their creative therapy practice outdoors or bring nature and her cycles into the clinic room and studio. In my mind's eye I see a new forest growing all over Britain, a forest of environmental arts therapy practice. But this is just the beginning, the gathering and planting of the seeds. This is the start of a new cycle, but no cycle stands alone for the seeds of the new are buried in the compost of the old.

The natural cycle of the turning year begins with the Celtic year in November when the autumn leaves lie crisp and golden upon the earth. But the leaves mark the end of the old cycle; it is that which they contain that holds the promise of the new.

Leaf mounds

It is a meeting of the Lionheart men's group, but one man sits alone, waiting in the dark woods on a damp November night. The leaves upon which he sits are cold and damp and all is silent. He has just turned off his head torch and only the faintest vestige of starlight filtering down through the branches above is allowing him to see anything at all. What he can just make out is that all around him, between the trees, are mysterious mounds of leaves. He is awed and stilled by their presence and feels almost as if he has stumbled across a prehistoric site and rests now among the graves of ancient chieftains. Some moments in our lives feel timeless and archetypal and this is such a moment. But these mounds are not of the past, this ritual is here and now, and they do not contain the dead for if the light allowed he would see them gently breathing.
For resting in the heart of every mound is a man.

Feeling is like a wild animal and may only come to us when we are still. So every ritual becomes a pause in the headlong gambol of our lives in which we allow ourselves to feel. Here we learn how the composting of our past feeds the seeds of our future. The cycle begins in November because now the trees choose wisely to plant their seeds in the compost of the old year. For this brief transition, the elder and the child lie together and are one. Often we make our inner children now sometimes tiny enough to place in match boxes and keep close to our hearts (Figure 1.1).

November is the first doorway of the year, but it leads into its dark half, into descent, for the seed must first lie dormant beneath the ground before it can begin to grow, a time of dreaming. So begins December, the lead up to the midwinter solstice, the deepest, darkest part of the year. Often we work indoors around a fire now; through visualisation we explore our own heart caves and the challenges and treasures to be found there. Or we venture outdoors where often the ice and the snow provide us with unsurpassable building materials for walls, dens, shrines, effigies and play.

In January the slow return of the sun gradually brings us to a point of balance stirring the dead land back into life. We often work with bridges and mobiles at this time, exploring our own balance between feeling and action. There comes a point of conception, usually towards the end of the month, when the balance tips and the seeds begin to awake.

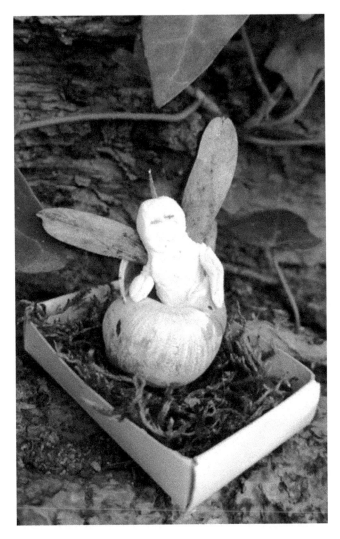

FIGURE 1.1   Child in matchbox

The seeds of my own environmental arts therapy practice grew from the composting of a much earlier time in my career, when I first moved my dramatherapy practice outdoors. From 1986 to 2001 I led a project called Daytime Community Therapies in Exeter, Devon, funded initially by Exeter Health Authority and then by Devon Partnership Trust. Daytime was a National Health Service (NHS) day service for adults with profound and complex disabilities and it hosted two outdoor projects: a carnival theatre company called Dreamtime Theatre and an outdoor activity programme called Naturesense.

Dreamtime Theatre built large carnival costumes and puppets, many of which were on wheelchairs, enabling adults with special needs to participate in community arts events. By combining disability arts with outdoor performance, it opened the studio door and allowed therapy to step outside. The stories that we performed were often improvised in story-making workshops and guided by nonverbal cues (facial expression, sound, movement and choices made by the participants). Many of these took place in the gardens or elsewhere in Devon, as part of Naturesense, a thrice weekly venture out into the wilds. By introducing our client group to outward bound or animal-based activity, environmental arts, storytelling and nature-based sensory activities, Naturesense furthered the process of moving outdoors. The bridge from one practice to the next came in the form of a secondment to the creative therapy unit on the floor above. This allowed me for the first time to take adult mental health service users out into the gardens for individual environmental arts therapy sessions.

Emerging

February begins with the ancient festival of Imbolc, meaning 'in the belly'. The ice is melting and feeling is returning to the land, and to ourselves. The soil becomes the soft moist womb and the seed within begins to grow. The life that we are living now is the womb that holds the new growth but there is often much feeling welling here, a need to let go of the old and leap into the new, and we often find ourselves in grief ritual at this time.

The womb

Geoff was a single man in his fifties who had never sustained a long-term relationship and was now concerned that he would never have children. He complained of being unable to find any feeling connection to women.

The therapist asked him about his mother and he said that she had died of a slow illness when he was a baby and he did not remember her. He was invited into the woods to find or make her there.

He stopped at a tree which, he said looked like the inverted body of a woman with her legs apart. He described this image as sexual and he felt ashamed for choosing it.

As he was looking around he noticed that someone else had made a little shrine in the hollow of a very old oak tree behind him. This, he said, was the opposite of the other tree, a sacred place of love, something that he had rarely felt. When the therapist reminded him that he had been mothered briefly, both in her womb and in her arms before she died, he began to cry. It seemed meaningful that this womb had been behind him all the time hidden in a distant and forgotten past.

He climbed back into the womb and spoke to his mother from five different places of feeling to unravel the strands of his grief.

He spoke to her from the place of fear, of being scared of the enduring impact of her leaving him, of not being able to trust to love.

He spoke to her from the place of guilt of his own sense of failure in relationships.

Then he spoke to her from the place of anger. He talked about her failure to set up loving care for him for after she had gone, even though her illness had been a slow one leaving him solely in the care of his inadequate and unemotional father. This, at last, was the true voice of his anger, raised and furious.

"You left me with him!"

Then he moved to the place of sadness and wept again for a long time until finally he could speak to his mother from the place of love. Then, within the hollow of the old oak, he made his own shrine for them both.

By March the new seedlings are emerging, pushing up from the soil like little spears. This masculine principle, this desire to push up and out, is strong in us all at this time and we often find ourselves on hillsides throwing spears of our own making, shouting our affirmations as we do so (see Figure 1.2).

In April we celebrate Easter, once the festival of Eostra (root of the word *oestrus*) the spring goddess. Her symbol was the egg and still we give eggs at this time. Now, when the buds in the trees are waiting to unfold and the eggs are waiting in the nest, this feeling of being born but not yet hatched is a common motif.

The eggs

Eli was a divorced woman in her thirties who complained of being bullied by her teenage son. She would not let herself get angry with him and when asked why, she said that she didn't want to be like her father who often lost his temper and hit her most days when she was a child.

She was invited into the woods to find or make her father.

She found an ivy clad fallen tree to represent him. She believed that he was an unhappy man who struggled with his life but kept all hidden until his temper broke.

As she talked about him she began to cry. She recalled how much she had loved him when she was little, how she would get up early to milk the

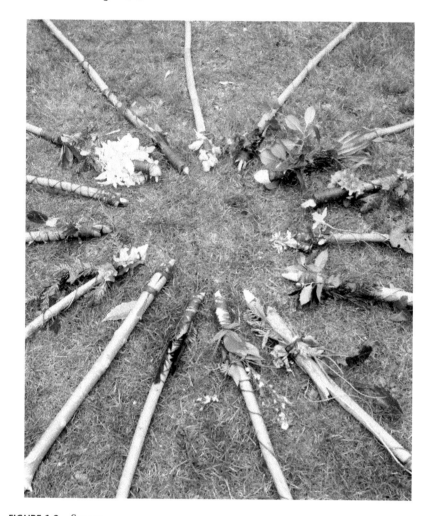

FIGURE 1.2 Spears

cows with him so that she had him to herself. They did not talk at these times, but he felt softer.

The therapist asked her to find something to represent her love and loyalty for her father and put it to one side where it would be safe. She chose a soft leaf and left it in another clearing nearby. The therapist explained that anything that was done would not impact on that love, that it was safe where she had put it.

She made an effigy of herself as a child and placed it in relation to her father. The therapist asked her to stand now as an adult and a parent *herself and consider the feelings of the child in relation to the father once the child's love for him had been taken out of the equation. She could see that the little girl was unheld, scared and frequently beaten and now felt her outrage at this. She shouted the words "I hate you!" over and over, louder and louder, ripping the ivy from the fallen tree, breaking off its branches and gouging out the rotten wood. As she did so she told him how his harsh fathering had compromised her ability to be in relationship with men and was now impacting on her relationship with her son. She continued until her anger was spent.*

In the humus of the rotten wood that she had pulled out, she began moulding six eggs. She said that they were her new beginnings and the therapist asked her to hold and name each one.

Then they returned to the child whom she gathered up and took away from her father. She found a soft bed for it in the arms of a fern and drew a line around it. They talked about how it feels when someone crosses that line and tramples on the soft heart within, and how important it was to use her anger to protect that boundary. This was especially so with her son, so that he learns how to respect her boundary and the boundary of others and then as an adult protect his own. They considered how her son's challenge was both a request for clarity regarding her boundary and an opportunity for her to practice giving it. This was the work that still needed to be done so that the eggs could hatch.

Working in the gardens of the creative therapy unit I began to notice how similar natural metaphors were appearing in my client's work at the same time. Seeking an indigenous frame of reference for this I found the Celtic Ogham tree calendar, an ancient system that relates one or more trees or plants to every month. Each tree has its own oracular meaning and medicine and seemed to be closely correlating with the spontaneously emerging metaphors. The Ogham tree alphabet and calendar first appeared in printed form in Robert O'Flaherty's *Ogygia* (1793), where it is presented as a genuine relic of druidism originally recorded in the medieval Irish manuscript *The Book of Lecan* written between 1397 and 1418 (O Cuirnin, 1397–1418). It was further examined by Robert Graves in *The White Goddess* (1948). I came across it in *The Celtic Tree Oracle: A System of Divination,* by Liz and Colin Murray (1988). As an oracular system it has found its home into modern paganism and esoteric literature and reappears in many different forms, some re-intuited. Consequently, it is hard to know what to trust.

For this reason I set up a research group called 'The Circle of Trees', offering free environmental arts therapy groupwork to anyone who would meet with me once a week for a year to explore the potential of this calendar in relation to working with their own unfolding personal process. We ended up a group of seven artists, therapists, storytellers and students. Over the year we improvised with new ways of working creatively outdoors, feeling into the connection between our own emotional journey and the metaphors offered by the calendar.

This group was so popular and so productive that we ran it again the following year with another body of participants, although this time fortnightly, as the weekly commitment was unsustainable. In fact, over the next seven years we ran it five times, at the end of which I had enough material to write the book *Environmental Arts Therapy and the Tree of Life*. This was not an academic book, neither was it a book solely for therapists. Poetic and practical, it sought to help anyone feel the connection between the turning of the year and the turning of their feelings. The release of this book was a further outreach of the research as it had to be read month by month, so that the content could be felt in context with the cycle and it contained an invitation for readers to email me and tell me about their experiences. Ten years on those emails are still flowing in and in my opinion there is now little doubt that the Ogham calendar is following our feeling journey through the year, here in these once Celtic lands. The Circle of Trees research group inspired me to begin a private environmental arts therapy practice working in local woodland with individual clients and groups. This ran alongside my NHS work and continues to this day.

Flowering

The festival of Beltane at the beginning of May is the second doorway of the year leading from the dark half to the light. Now comes the great green tidal wave of spring unfurling from below and tumbling down from above. So begins the most solar and masculine time of the year with the gathering of power in May and its expression in June. The land becomes a pressure cooker and we all cook together, so this a time when anger and empowerment work often come to the fore.

Two effigies

Lucy was a woman in her thirties who complained of being unable to trust her own judgement or opinion. She lived with a female flatmate who constantly challenged and judged her, making her question herself. The therapist asked her to trace this distrust back to its source and she arrived at her mother. They sought to find or make her in the woods.

Lucy stopped at a holly tree, which she described as the "tree of sacrifice". She said that her mother had lived such a life dedicating her time to looking after her husband and seven children. As she shared about her childhood the therapist felt her ambivalence so asked her to make two effigies, one for the positive mothering that she had received and one for the negative. First they approached the positive, which leant tall and spindly with open arms against a rotten stump.

She reflected on how resilient and resourceful her mother had been to raise so many children in a time of lack. She spoke of how welcoming and hospitable she had been to others, although she felt that these open arms were just for show and were never extended to her or her siblings. She felt no love in this place, only admiration for her mother's strength and endurance in the face of her own disappointments.

The negative mothering clambered over a fallen oak tree like an ugly spider. Immediately it was evident from her tears that there was more feeling here and she began to tell the story of the time when in old age her mother had accused her of stealing from her. She admitted with some embarrassment how she and her siblings did steal from their mother when they were young, money from her purse and cigarettes too, and that consequently her mother had never trusted any of them. But to be accused of this as an adult when it was not true and when she had given so much of her time to care for her mother in old age had been deeply hurtful. She spoke to her mother about this now and wept. The therapist asked her to consider to what extent she had integrated her mother's distrust into her own sense of self. She felt that this was true and, feeling her anger, smashed up the ugly spider and threw the pieces into the woods. Immediately she began to express her distrust at whether she had just done the right thing or not, so the therapist asked her to gather up again the big stick that had run through the heart of the ugly spider like a spine and to deal with it once and for all. She said that she wanted to break it against the fallen tree. She tried, quite weakly at first, but then harder and harder until she was weeping, remembering her own beatings at the hands of her mother. Only then, as she roared her anguish, did she muster enough force to break the stick.

Then she made an effigy of the child that she had been and took it to another place. She put it in the bole of an ash, held safely between three strong boughs. The therapist told her how traditionally the ash is the tree of alchemy, transmuting the lead of our wounding into the gold of our personal growth. She was asked to touch and feel into each of the three boughs to see what it was that she had created out of her wounding. In this way she honoured her own strengths of character.

This build-up of power reaches its zenith in the midsummer solstice, after which we spill back down into the stillness of the feminine in July. Here we may begin to feel the deep undercurrents that underlay our conflicts like a dark pool. This dark pool, the cauldron of the unconscious, is a common metaphor here and often when we begin to feel into it, we find shame waiting.

Homunculus

John was a man in his sixties who struggled to maintain an academic reputation in the face of his depression, self-doubt and anxiety.

He was climbing through the branches of a fallen tree and was drawn to a strong earthy smell and scrabbled in the soil under the branches, emerging with a handful of pungent humus. He and his therapist reflected together: humus, human, humiliation, humility. He squashed it into a little human shape, a homunculus.

"This is my shame" he said and as he spoke the therapist noticed him touch his big round belly. "Is it in there?" they asked.

He considered and then replied, "Yes I think that it has always been in here".

Holding the little earthen child to his belly he felt into his beginnings. He spoke of being born to a mother who was too unwell at the time to hold him and never did again, of their bonding falling by the wayside, a lost opportunity never to be reclaimed. He imagined his belly still swelling, reaching still for the lost umbilicus, the last loving connection to mother.

"This is the shame baby" he said. He held it in his hand but could not feel the child's suffering. It was before words, there were no words, only the guessing in retrospect, imagining how the child must have felt. A feeling message to a brand new heart: you are not worth loving. And still that message enduring always at the core of him.

The child was tiny, but the therapist could feel the weight of his shame and asked him if they might help him bear it. They leant him a hand. Only when they bore the child together did he begin to weep.

He made a little nest for the homunculus and covered it in leaves. "I see you now" he said. As he put his hand protectively over the child, he swore that he felt its tiny hand touch him back.

He returned to this place again when he was struggling with a sense of his own inadequacy having been offered a prestigious academic opportunity. On this occasion he remembered being a boy at school hiding among the lockers from the bullies, hunted and alone. Climbing into the branches he imagined that boy paralysed with fear among the brambles below. Weeping now, he spoke down to him as if he was his own guardian angel, comforting him, reassuring him that they would be ok and that only by this rite of passage could this boy become this man. He left feeling lighter, clearer, stronger. By bringing shame to the surface John had turned it into a place of personal resource and empowerment.

In 2001 I moved fully into mental health services to set up the Wild Things project, which ran out of Russell Clinic, a centre for recovery and independent living services in Wonford House Hospital in Exeter, funded by Devon Partnership Trust. Based loosely on Naturesense and drawing together many of the same service providers, Wild Things offered a comprehensive programme of outward-bound activity, animal-assisted therapies, bushcraft, storytelling and environmental arts therapy. It was aimed mainly at young men who had been given a diagnosis of schizophrenia or drug induced psychosis, a client group who had been previously very difficult to engage, often preferring to spend their time smoking or listening to music rather than attend the hospital activity centre. But when we appeared offering to take them quad biking, abseiling, kayaking or llama walking, motivational levels changed.

Many of these young men stayed on the clinic for a year or more. Because they were coming out with us several times a week and we were all getting to know each other on the end of a rope, around a camp fire or in a wobbly canoe, relationships based on trust, camaraderie and shared achievement blossomed and paved the way for individual environmental arts therapy. Although this could and did take any shape, it very soon acquired recognition within the multi-disciplinary team as a place to refer clients with anger related issues. Before long many young men were coming into the woods either because they were trying and failing to repress anger that desperately needed release or because they could not access their anger and so were defenseless and easily abused by others. Here they could make and break, shout and scream, and connect often for the first time to the feelings that lay beneath. But when these young men were discharged the service stopped and there was little in the community to compare, so leaving the hospital became for some a backward step. In response we set up Wild Things In The Community in partnership with Mind in Exeter, the mental health charity, offering a wide variety of outdoor activities and compiling a directory of these that service users could use themselves. This meant that when an individual with our support had found an activity that they loved they could work out how to access it independently in their own time and at their own cost. Wild Things In The Community was a non-therapeutic programme that offered opportunity and education and it radically changed people's expectations about what life had to offer them.

Fruiting

August begins with the festival of Lammas, marking the first harvest. The orchards are abundant with swelling and fragrant fruit and nuts and berries cluster among the hedgerows while the wild vines wrap themselves around all. Everywhere now the vegetation is overgrown and running to seed and although this is a time when we can connect deeply to our own emotional and practical harvest, we can also begin to feel overwhelmed now as if we are bearing the weight of the world.

This is the dark harvest, the chaff that must be blown away to reveal the good grain, and we often make masks at this time to show who we become when the dark harvest overwhelms us or make a yoke to carry our burdens until we can throw them down in anger.

In September the outward push of summer comes to an end and the hedgerows hang heavy with blackberries, elderberries and sloes, the dark fruit of the feminine. Now in the autumnal retreat we begin to spiral back into ourselves and as we do so we meet whatever still blocks us, the shadow waiting for us to own and address it. The hedgerows are full of spiders' webs too at this time, sparkling in the low autumn sun and we also can feel trapped and held fast as we confront these barriers within ourselves.

The wall

Patrick was a man in his thirties. He spoke about entering his current relationship with a son from the one before and how his current partner had at first been supportive and accepting of this, but then when a child was born to them both she had spurned the first. He spoke of his fury at this, how he had felt betrayed, how it had exploded into acts of near violence and scared them both. Such rage was a new experience for him as he had always been passive and as a child quiet and obedient.

He was invited into the woods to look for or make that child. He found a safe shady place at the foot of an oak tree and made a little figure from sticks and leaves. He talked about being a baby. He knew that his mother had breast fed him so he must have been held as an infant, but he could not remember her holding him later, only judging and shaming him. He named the little child figure as "the death of trust" and wept in this place.

The therapist asked him about the oak tree. He said that it was the beanstalk waiting for Jack to climb it. All that Jack had needed was affirmation from others, encouragement, love and support, but that had never been forthcoming, so he had never climbed. The child was still there, still waiting for the adventure to begin.

The therapist asked him to find whatever had been there in the place of those things. He found a scrubby little hawthorn to describe the parenting that he had received. The therapist told him that traditionally the hawthorn is a tree of love, associated with the opening of heart. But this one was almost void of leaves baring only its thorns. It was sad to behold, and here he felt his empathy for his parents talking about the poor parenting that they had received themselves.

The therapist asked him to name the spirit that ran as a legacy across the generations blighting his parent's life and his own and threatening his children now. He called it "fear" and started to make it.

He made a huge wall of ivy, roots and branches in the crook of a tree, twisted, gnarled and camouflaged, trying to stay hidden but still blocking the path. When he was asked how he felt about this he grinned and said "I know where this is heading. You want me to smash it up, but the fact is its a place of comfort for me, it feels safe."

"Keep it then" replied the therapist.

"Oh I don't know if I like that" he said.

He began to see that he was choosing to continue the parental legacy, keeping his inner child down by judging and shaming himself, keeping his anger muted until it was on a hair trigger, feeling his own betrayal in the rejection of his son. His anger at the wall that he had built for himself was beginning to smoulder now so the therapist asked him to speak out loud one angry word that described it.

"Cage" he said.

He was asked to say it again, but this time so loud that the whole forest would hear.

"Cage" he roared over and over again and he kicked and smashed the wall breaking every branch and root against the trees until every part of it was completely destroyed.

Then he stood in the doorway that he had cleared. The therapist asked him to name what lay on the other side and he called it 'freedom'. He stood on the threshold, knowing both cage and freedom and that he had a choice

October brings the end of the year's cycle, concluding with the festival of Samhain or Hallow'een when it was traditionally believed that our ancestors stand nearest to us. The old leaves are falling and death is all around us and within us too. This is the time when we honour our elders and the elders within ourselves. But in every ending there is a beginning and like reeds bending in the river's current we begin now to feel the pull of the new cycle.

Reed boats

It is the closing ceremony of the postgraduate certificate course. One by one each participant is clothed in the robe of the elder, given their certificate and honoured for their passage through the year, a journey of feeling, sharing and learning. The day before we had been working near the water and all had made beautiful reed boats for themselves, placing in each natural symbols of all that they were affirming now for the cycle to come, the seeds of their future. Each now holds their boat upon their lap and shares the meaning of its cargo.

After the ceremony we all walk through the crowds of Kings Cross carrying the boats down to the canal to launch them. How mysterious and incongruous they seem, paraded in this manner through the streets of inner-city London. I am often asked why we teach environmental arts therapy here instead of in the countryside where we would be spoilt for locations to work in. But if our students can learn it here, they can take it anywhere (see Figure 1.3).

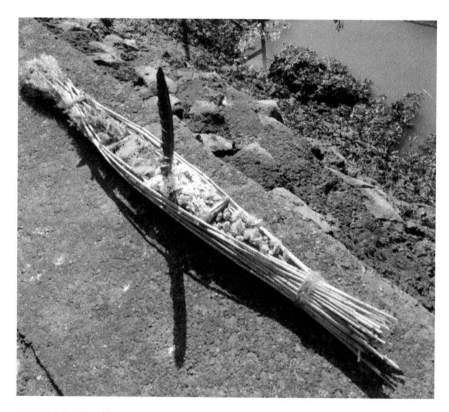

FIGURE 1.3 Reed boat

The move from Devon to London began when Gary Nash visited Wild Things In The Community, having read an article on grief that I had written for *Resurgence* magazine (Siddons Heginworth 2010). From that meeting initially came seasonal environmental arts therapy workshops at the London Art Therapy Centre and then in 2013 the first postgraduate certificate course. Open only to qualified creative therapists (art, drama, music or dance/movement), the course helps its trainees to take their practice outdoors and work in relationship with the turning year. It runs every two years and consequently there is now a growing population of practicing environmental arts therapists in Britain, many of whom are contributing to this book. This is a book about beginnings, because many of the contributors have only just begun taking their practice outdoors or bringing nature in. But each is a pathfinder daring to open the clinic room doors and follow metaphor and feeling into the trees and wherever it leads them, intrepid scouts in the wild frontiers of the heart.

In the summer of 2018 the first ever gathering of environmental arts therapists at Holbeam Woods in Devon led to the creation of Environmental Arts Therapy UK. Its aims are to grow and promote environmental arts therapy, organise twice yearly gatherings and provide continued professional development events for its members. Meanwhile there are now four more Circle of Trees groups, one in London, one in Essex, one in Edinburgh and another in Hertfordshire. So, as in all turning, we spiral round to where we began and find ourselves grown.

But here at the close, do we not also feel death all around us? Many of the contributors to this book reflect upon the role that environmental arts therapy can play in responding to the environmental crisis, for we can no longer consider our therapeutic journeys in isolation (as if truly we ever could). Environmental arts therapy emerges now out of a deep longing for reconnection and serves this process in many ways. Firstly it gives us a means to raise income from the land in a manner that is best served wholly by leaving it alone and allowing it to run wild. Secondly it facilitates a deep personal connection between soul and soil, between the individual in therapy and the landscape in which the therapy takes place, for the conversation between both is deeply personal and always leads to the love of one for the other. Thirdly, and perhaps of most importance, it allows us to feel our part in the great wounding of the Earth, not just as perpetrators but as victims, for we are only doing outwardly to nature what has been done to ourselves. Generations of us have been raised in a culture that promotes and idolises the active masculine and neglects and shames the feeling feminine. The consequences of this are all invasive, impacting on everything that requires integrity of heart: the manner in which we raise our children, the means by which we initiate our young (or don't), the way that we respond to ill health, the way that we honour elders (or not), the way that we interact with and misuse the natural world and, most insidious of all, the way that we are encouraged to numb, avoid and distract from feeling within ourselves. This cultural neglect of the feminine, both outwardly with nature and inwardly with the feeling self, has left us all deforested, polluted and ailing.

Perhaps only when we take climate change personally will we really be able to assist in its turning.

References

Avinoam, N. (2002). The fertilization dance: A mechanical view of the egg rotation during the initial spermatozoa-ovum interaction. Academic Press. National Center for Biotechnology Information, U.S. National Library of Medicine. *Journal of Theoretical Biology*, 214 (2), pp. 171–179.

Davies, J. (1999). Environmental art therapy: Metaphors in the field. *The Arts in Psychotherapy*, 26 (4), pp. 45–49.

Graves, R. (1948). *The white goddess: A historical grammar of poetic myth*. London: Faber & Faber.

Murray, L., and Murray, C. (1988). *The Celtic tree oracle, a system of divination*. London: Connections Book Publishing.

O Cuirnin, A. (1397–1418). *The (Great) Book of Lecan (Irish: Leabhar (Mór) Leacain)*. Royal Irish Academy.

O'Flaherty, R. (1684). *Ogygia, or a chronological account of Irish events*. W. M'kenzie, translated by Hely, J. (1793). Reprinted by Forgotten Books (2018).

Siddons Heginworth, I. (2008). *Environmental arts therapy and the tree of life*. Exeter: Spirits Rest Books.

Siddons Heginworth, I. (2010). Unlocking the grief. *Resurgence*, July/August, Issue 261.

Siddons Heginworth, I., Kaplan, H., and Nash, G. (2013). *Environmental arts therapy course handbook*. London: London Art Therapy Centre.

2

WEAVING THE THREADS OF THEORY AND EXPERIENCE

A review of the literature

Gary Nash

Introduction

In weaving the threads of theory and experience I will draw together a review of the literature in the areas of ecopsychology, ecotherapy and taking the creative arts therapies outdoors. The aim of this review is firstly to provide an evidence-based and referenced context through which the emergence of nature-informed therapies can be understood, whilst locating these developments within a well-considered theoretical and practice-based structure. Secondly it considers how environmental arts therapy is emerging from an integrative creative arts approach in which all the arts are bought into play when working therapeutically out of doors. It is important to note that the clinical contexts in which the creative arts therapies are practiced and their development within healthcare and education here in Britain will also continue to shape emerging theories, methods and approaches to clinical practice. This review will therefore also consider some of the challenges and opportunities we face when the therapeutic frame is radically altered by taking the work of therapy outside.

Ecology, ecopsychology and ecotherapies

Ecopsychology is the name often used for the emerging synthesis of psychological and ecological disciplines. Roszak's (1995) initial vision for ecopsychology sought to place the psyche back in context with the earth, arguing that "life and mind emerge via evolution within an unfolding sequence of the physical, biological, mental and cultural systems" (Roszak, 1992, p. 132). "Ecopsychology proceeds from the assumption that at its deepest level the psyche remains sympathetically bonded to the earth that mothered it into existence" (Roszak, 1995, p. 5). Roszak proposes that the core of mind is the ecological unconscious – a place where our inherent reciprocity and connection to the natural world exists at the centre of our being. The umbrella term for the application of ecopsychology in a clinical context is ecotherapy.

Ecotherapy represents a new form of psychotherapy that acknowledges the vital role of nature and addresses the human – nature relationship (Buzzell and Chalquist, 2009; Roszak, 2009). The emergence of the term 'ecotherapy' and 'ecopsychology' over the past 30 years provides a conceptual framework from which to view the self in relation to acting within, being acted upon, being shaped and influenced by, the living world. The application of theory in this area has led to a description of practice from a range of therapists, counsellors and psychotherapists who have taken their work out of doors. Several authors (Jordan, 2009, 2012, Jones et al., 2016; Dodds, 2012; Totton, 2011; Rust and Totton, 2012) consider environmental processes of ecology and our total dependence upon natural systems with reference to existing psychological, developmental and relational theories.

Psychotherapist and academic Martin Jordan (2012) wrote about the relationship between psychotherapy and the wider cultural and political sphere and the interaction between our environment, mental health and well-being. Jordan widens our understanding of human-nature relatedness and raises the problem of subjective interiors and objective material exteriors, considering how they meet, connect, relate and communicate: "The starting point for understanding human-nature relations leaves us with the problem of how subjective interiors and objective material exteriors come into some form of communication" (Jordan, 2012, p. 139). Our conceptual understanding of this inter-connection between internal experience and external relating is central to the processes of communication within a psychotherapeutic dyadic relationship. Jordan helps us to think about the continuum that exists when we diminish the separations we place between ego, self, other and nature and begin to experience ourselves in a relational flow between self, other and place.

The importance of identifying a reciprocal process whereby healing in nature is also healing for nature is highlighted by art therapist and Jungian analyst Rust (2012). She asks us to consider deep questions within our work as art psychotherapists such as: what can the study of natural systems (ecology) teach us about human systems and how do the wider issues of global crisis and our relationship with nature come into the therapy relationship? Rust (2012) proposes a need to listen to the 'earth stories' we each hold within, viewing them as being of equal important to our human stories of love, loss and attachment styles. Drawing on the earth-based wisdom of indigenous peoples and of rites of passage work, Rust works outdoors in wilderness settings as well as woodland spaces in North London.

Nurturing a reciprocal relationship

The dynamic flow of conscious and unconscious feeling and affect move through the experiences we have in our bodies and in relationship with the other, one's client. How we theorise this dynamic shapes our practice and therapeutic approach.

The conceptual frame we use to hold and channel this process enables us to feel and be affected by the client's nonverbal flow of feeling and inner experience. As we do so we facilitate this movement of energy in order to benefit the client's self-awareness and emotional health. Our understanding of this reciprocal flow between self and other is a cornerstone of psychodynamic thought and therapeutic process and is of central importance for the creative arts therapies.

In *Art as Medicine* (1992) McNiff describes the healing qualities of the creative process as a reciprocal flow between self and image as one creates. He describes the process whereby an artist or artist/therapist and, by extension, a client in therapy, engages with image-making, deepening into a physical experience, and emerging to reflect on the art piece. We do this time and time again as we lose ourselves and find something of ourselves in the creative act. More recently McNiff (2016) describes the healing energies of art as being an "ecological process of creativity" and a vital circulation of creative energies: "The healing process of creativity corresponds to the ecological forces of nature – an open-ended 'ecology of imagination' – creative expression encouraging infinitely variable processes of expression" (McNiff, 2016, p. 473).

Atkins and Snyder (2018) include reciprocity in their definition of Nature-based expressive arts therapy. They see reciprocity as our mutual interdependence between humans and the earth and refer to Guattari (2000) who defined the 'three ecologies' as being the "circular relationship between environmental – mental – and social ideologies or 'mind, nature and society'" (Atkins and Snyder, 2018, p. 55). The reciprocal flow of energy experienced within a nature-therapist-client relationship extends and develops this principle still further as Nature holds and supports both therapist and client in the work. Our understanding of the potential to work with the naturally occurring ecological forces of nature plays a central role in shaping a practitioner's methods and approach when we move our work outdoors.

Introducing environmental arts therapy

Emerging from the field of the creative arts therapies

The creative arts therapies have long developed an awareness and engagement with the presence and influence of nature in clinical practice. Nature is sometimes presented by clients through the use of metaphor and imagery in the studio. Images of trees, views, landscapes and inscapes are imagined and painted or modelled using traditional art materials. Natural materials may also be bought into session and used as metaphors or integrated into the art-making process. The image of trees as 'symbolic of self' have been recorded by art therapist Camilla Connell (1998) in relation to her work with patients with a terminal or life threatening illness. The emergence of the image of singular trees in clients' images are linked to certain transitions in nature. When confronted with terminal illness the symbol of the tree tends to connects us to something in one's nature that seems: "stronger and more sustainable than a physical ailing body, something that perhaps can be subject to transformation" (Connell, 1998, p. 98). Hephzibah Kaplan (2019) has collated 90 images of trees under the heading 'draw yourself as a tree' showing how people respond to the invitation to imagine the connection between self and nature and the powerful associations people have with trees in particular.

The first published use of the term 'environmental art therapy' was used by art therapist Jean Davies in her paper "Environmental Art Therapy: Metaphors from the Field" (1999). Davies describes her instructions to the first art therapy group to go 'off-site' 'scavenging' for materials for the making of a sculpture park in an old and derelict plot of land within an urban environment. The encounter with outdoors is described through an imaginative dialogue between group participants where both the land and the psychological fears, projections and fantasies that the space triggered are explored. She describes the therapeutic process which emerged from the 'scavenger hunt' with the group:

> Once patterns are discovered a space can open for clients to play with the metaphors which have arisen, allowing for ways in which to work with underlying issues through a less threatening object. An example of this is the empty lot that surrounded us – it was once a home.
>
> *(Davies, 1999, p. 46)*

Davies continues to develop her practice and her most recent paper entitled "Drawing Nature" invites us to connect with and "truly see and experience the continual change that is nature" (Davies, 2017, p. 66). Davies encourages us to take our arts practice outside and to work with beauty and resistance, longing and disappointment, experiencing the vitality of one's body in nature and channelling this energy into the art-making process. She describes how taking an attentive, observing position, one can experience the gradual, subtle, immediate or sudden changes in light, shadow, temperature or movement; if we attune to them, they give us a sense of our own movements, moods and shifts in temperament: "Observing and moving with change allows us to practice getting more comfortable with change and, thereby, practicing being fully awake" (Davies, 2017, p. 66). In this way Davies shows us that being outside in natural environments stirs our senses and wakes us up to what is around us and, in a reciprocal exchange of vital energy, we wake up to our own internal physiological and psychological energies.

In *Eco-art Therapy: Creative activities that let the Earth teach* Sweeney (2013) adds an arts-based perspective to the growing research in working therapeutically in and with Nature. She combines art therapy with immersion in nature whilst also drawing on an older knowledge of the earth which derives from indigenous cultures. As a practical guide to working therapeutically in nature Sweeny provides a framework which I summarise as follows: initially framing the therapy session with a focus upon a particular aspect of nature that one is naturally attracted to, then working with intent upon that attraction. The therapy process encourages an exploration of this attraction with words and also a sensory exploration; this is followed by an art response to the feelings aroused by this attraction, and finally: "using the visual expression to help you translate your enjoyable sensory experience into words so that you can think with it" (Sweeney, 2013, p. 17). This graduated and focused process provides a structure for working outdoors therapeutically, particularly in groups, and is explored further in the work of Jones et al (2016) and Kopytin and Rugh (2016, 2017).

Art therapist Jones (Jones et al., 2016) describes working outdoors within an adult National Health Service (NHS) art therapy provision using common land opposite the hospital grounds in an urban setting. Jones uses a combination of mindful-meditation practice, aware walking and sensory exercise, leading into a creative response in the form of art-making with found objects and natural materials. The movement into the landscape and into art-making is described as a structured process held by two facilitators. The transition into creative art-making is an invitation for group members to touch, to play and to respond to the experience of whatever is happening within themselves and whatever they sense around them in the space:

> Art work made outdoors can be built around, within or on top of living things. They can be placed in considered ways within the surrounding landscape, giving a further dimension for personal and group discovery through the power of grounding our internal experience and sharing this with others.
>
> *(Jones et al., 2016, p. 168)*

Art-making is followed by reflection on the experience, a closing circle, and the walk back to the clinical setting.

Outdoor music therapy

Eric Pfeifer (2017) describes Outdoor Music Therapy (OdMT) as an emerging practice which seeks to find safe and appropriate outdoor locations in which to experience the rhythm and textures of sound within a music therapy framework. He describes outdoor locations such as underground car parks, mountain huts, caves, sports halls and forests as offering potential to work with voice, body and melody. He suggests that taking music therapy outdoors has an influence on the therapeutic process: "There is movement, development, expression and extension, metamorphosis, modulation, growth – in other words something is evolving and changing, music therapy is not the same" (Pfeifer, 2017, p. 185).

In relation to bringing nature indoors Pfeifer describes the use of 'nature recordings' to attune the listener to a natural soundscape. Sounds of nature can evoke an imaginative response to the spaces that one can hear in the recording, they can also be used to accompany a relaxation process or to engage with the memories evoked. Mimicking, finding a melody or a beat in the playback recordings, may also lead to developing improvised themes. The sounds of nature and the spaces and places in and around us are diverse and multi-layered: "Imagine the steady change of the seasons, the regular shift from dawn to dusk, the continuous flowing of a river, the enduring sound of breaking sea waves. . . . There is movement and stillness, ritual and tradition, continuity and recurring change." (Pfeifer, 2017, p. 188)

Dramatherapy: nature therapy

Dramatherapist Ronen Berger (2009, 2014, 2016, 2017) has drawn together concepts and methods from dramatherapy and shamanism and combined them into what he has described as "Nature Therapy" (Berger, 2014). Berger identifies a central term which reflects the themes of reciprocity and our physical senses, he places an emphasis on the tactile sense and 'touching nature' becomes an underpinning concept in his approach which is shared by Davies (2017). According to Berger nature also calls for playfulness and connects us to our inner child and our creativity. In this approach metaphors and physical-sensory experiences with nature are believed to: "help the individual experience the world through additional perspectives, undergo recovery processes, and create a preferred alternative reality" (Berger, 2017, p. 52). Berger has developed this approach working in areas affected by conflict and has worked with children and communities suffering from the effects of war (2016). The methods and approaches developed have a direct relevance for working with clients experiencing trauma and loss.

Nature-based and expressive arts therapies

> This approach strives to achieve well-being and multiple treatment goals for individuals, families and communities and promote sustainable styles of life through people's involvement in expressive and creative activities in relation to environments in which they live.
>
> *(Kopytin and Rugh, 2017, p. 1)*

This description of Nature-based therapies is given by Kopytin and Rugh (2017) linking creative arts therapies and working outdoors with the emerging field of the expressive arts therapies movement. As leading academics and practitioners in the field their first publication, *The Green Studio* (2016), invited the art therapies to develop its own innovative and creative responses to working with nature as co-therapist in outdoor studios, nature specific landscapes and open-air therapeutic contexts. Kopytin (2016) and Berger (2016) both write about the importance of finding the right space and providing structured therapeutic activity. Kopytin (2017) describes how the term 'green studio' was introduced to define a special place where eco-arts therapeutic sessions can take place. These spaces are described as accessible green areas in the grounds of an institution or community setting: "it is a place which is made special" (Kopytin, 2017, p. 42). Kopytin and Rugh (2016, 2017) have furthered the theoretical scope of nature-based and nature-assisted therapies combining the arts. Their recent work integrates their theoretical perspectives within an integrative creative arts framework which is aligned with the 'expressive arts therapies'.

Atkins and Snyder (2018) also describe their work within the expressive arts therapies highlighting how the International Expressive Arts Therapy Association continues to form deep connections with ecology through their biennial conference focus on the arts therapies and the Earth (Atkins and Snyder, 2018, p. 47). In their book the authors present a thorough and detailed review of the existing literature in the area of the arts, ecological sciences and indigenous cultures. They examine the connections between the arts and our relationship with creativity, they elaborate our understanding of how we are connected to the natural cycles and ecosystems, and they also consider an older wisdom of attunement and ritual. They highlight the importance of reciprocity and resilience when we live, work and create in mutually sustainable relationships with the Earth (Atkins and Snyder, 2018, p. 55).

Environmental arts therapy

Siddons Heginworth (2008) describes the practice of environmental arts therapy as working with natural materials in natural environments through the unfolding year. Drawing on the use of metaphor and synchronicity his approach is focused on the personal and internal reflections of self that we find mirrored in the environments around us. *Environmental Arts Therapy and the Tree of Life* (2008) offers a framework for working through deep personal obstacles, blocks and struggles which, mirrored in the changing aspects of nature, encourage us to see our wounds reflected and transform them within the safety of natural landscapes. The use of symbolism and metaphor is central to his approach as is the exploration and elaboration of the reciprocal relationship between the individual and the earth. The practice of environmental arts therapy, as described in the book, shows how nature brings us to a visual, physical and symbolic encounter with the self, and more particularly, with the unconscious part of oneself which is stirred and activated by what we find in our encounters there.

In 2013 Siddons Heginworth delivered the first postgraduate one-year course in environmental arts therapy, held at The London Art Therapy Centre. The course combines integrative arts media, mythopoeic narratives and therapeutic processes in order to facilitate a heightened experience of self in relation to that which we make in our art outdoors or find reflected back at us in nature. The most succinct definition of environmental arts therapy is taken from the one-year certificated course handbook:

> Environmental arts therapy is the therapeutic use of natural materials, natural locations, natural themes and natural cycles. As in all arts therapy the therapeutic goals are the same however the context and references are drawn from the natural world, using myths and metaphors that relate to the time of year and the geographical and cultural location within which the therapy takes place.
>
> *(Siddons Heginworth et al., 2013, p. 2)*

The cultural stories and myths used to underpin the course material derive from an indigenous source found in the Celtic Ogham tree calendar which places one or more specific trees in each month of the year. The influence of trees upon written language is evidenced by Celtic artefacts that show a direct link between cypher marks used to represent particular trees and the same marks used to form the early Irish alphabet or Ogham (Graves, 1948). During the course this knowledge is elaborated with reference to stories, rituals and myths drawn from Celtic and worldwide traditions. This approach offers us an understanding of the relationship between the internal process of the individual, the turning year and an archetypal knowledge found in these older cultural narratives.

Within indigenous Celtic culture seasonal changes are marked by festivals which occur at significant points in the year. The cycle begins with the festival of Samhain, leading us into November and the descent into the 'dark half' of the year. Imbolc in early February marks the first stirring of life, followed by the spring equinox. Beltane at the beginning of May marks the movement into the 'light half' of the year, leading us to the summer solstice. Lughnasadh (Lammas) marks the harvest in August, to be followed by the autumn equinox, with the year ending in October. Many of these festivals are accompanied by indigenous cultural stories drawn from Celtic source material (Patterson, 1996; Gifford, 2000). A rich source of scientific, cultural and historic material which complements this work can be found in Hageneder's *The Spirit of Trees* (2000) and *The Heritage of Trees* (2001). He considers how people, communities and cultures have related to trees as natural forces, developing a reliance and deep interconnection on their potential to provide shelter, food, fuel and healing. Our dependency and interrelationship led to the use of trees and plants for medicinal purposes and the emergence of symbolic qualities which have been woven into ancient and worldwide mythologies.

Challenges and opportunities when moving therapy outdoors

Therapeutic frames, boundaries and thresholds

When training to become a therapist the conceptual and ethical foundation of professional practice rest upon the requirement of a private, clearly defined clinical space. This is a space which is uninterrupted, protected, cared for, reliable and consistent. The emphasis upon safety and confidentiality provides a stable inner frame within which the work of therapy can take place. The concrete spaces we use become synonymous in our thinking with 'holding' and 'containing' the metaphoric and internal spaces we explore in the therapy relationship. Moving outdoors challenges our assumptions about the spaces we use and also our reliance upon the built environment. These challenges refer to the symbolic and conceptual framework which we internalise as therapists, as well as the practical problems associated with relocation.

Nick Totton (2012) refers to the therapeutic 'frame' and 'boundaries' as being spatial terms that we use to conceptualise how we behave within them. In the psychological work of therapy we use these terms to 'hold' and 'contain' the thoughts, feelings, fantasies and projections that our clients bring to the work. The spatial concept creates in our mind a picture of "objective edges or thresholds which can be objectively crossed or not crossed, erased or preserved" (Totton, 2012, p. 261). Art therapist Schaverien (1989) in her chapter, The Picture within the Frame, defines the 'inner' and 'outer' frame in art therapy. The 'outer frame' describes the context and the organisational setting in which the work takes place and refers to the "boundaries around the physical space including the time and the limits of therapy" (Schaverien, 1989, p. 148). The outer frame is the clinical context and the boundaries within the care setting or institution that support the work of therapy. The 'inner frame' refers to the therapist's conscious attention and attitude towards the client, the picture and the art-making within the triangular relationship in art therapy. The practice of environmental arts therapy, along with other nature-based therapies, uses an approach that is located and held within a wider environmental frame situated outside; this poses a challenge to the conventional view of therapy.

Through the development of the portable studio Kalmanowitz and Lloyd (1997, 2005) showed that art therapy can be used effectively out of doors in wars zones where the built environment is structurally unsafe or a potential target and also effectively in their work with refugees or in the aftermath of natural disasters. They demonstrate however that art therapy in these contexts is not just about taking art materials outside, it is also about stepping out of the clinical setting, buildings, and institutions and engaging with the social and cultural realities which people, one's clients, inhabit. They found that the challenge presented by a traumatised/unpredictable outer frame is not insurmountable and demonstrate how art therapists can carry the inner frame of psychodynamic thinking with them and transpose this onto their work with clients when working outdoors.

The psychodynamic frame linked to our knowledge of developmental psychology and the theories, methods and approaches we use to facilitate a creative response with our clients can, from this perspective, be taken out of the consulting room. In so doing we find that we relax our reliance upon the literal concrete frames that we establish for our practice and begin to see them as Milner (1957) sees them – "as conceptual frames, bracketing time and space, separating what happens within the frame of the therapy hour from what happened before and after that hour" (Milner, 1957, p. 152). As creative arts therapists, when we step outside we are required to cross this conceptual threshold and, in so doing, we must question the assumptions that we hold and have been trained to maintain. What is emerging is an opening up of the tight and clear, human-made concrete boundaries and clinical spaces provided by conventional therapy practice.

Nature becomes the 'outside frame'

If we consider nature as holding the therapeutic process beyond the outer frame of the institution we can begin to consider how therapist, client and nature might experience each other and interact with therapeutic intention. This may include seeing nature as 'co-therapist' (Pfeifer, 2017) or 'active partner' (Berger, 2016). The way we perceive this relationship is important to the development of facilitation approach, methods and technique. According to Pfeifer the creative arts therapy dyadic relationship is mediated through the arts, methods, media and materials and this produces what we know as the triangular relationship with the arts representing the third relational position. Pfeifer describes how nature "favourably changes and affects this system" (Pfeifer, 2017, p. 187). Nature becomes an active partner in the therapeutic relationship: "The therapist sets the framework allowing the patient to get closer contact with him/herself and the natural environment – and to carefully assist the emerging process" (Pfeifer, 2017, p. 187). Nature also acts as a container for the therapeutic work, as observer of the work and provider of materials.

The relationship between therapist, client and environment is described as a focus of attention by Martin Jordan: "*Therapy expands to include both the therapeutic dyad and the third space of nature, which either forms a backdrop to the therapy or situates itself in the foreground of the work, taking the form of powerful metaphors and symbols*" (Jordan and Hinds, 2016, p. 66).

Berger (2016) explains how nature is an active partner in the therapeutic relationship, unlike the artwork in the triangular relationship: "Nature plays its own role, having an intrinsic value with a life and dynamic of its own" (Berger, 2016, p. 178). From this perspective Berger views nature as a presence in the therapeutic process which informs the practitioner's approach and positioning in relation to the client's process. The therapist can take a central role in the interaction with the client so that nature is in the background. Alternatively "the therapist can take a secondary position as a mediator between the client and nature by being a witness to a process occurring directly with nature" (Berger, 2017, p. 50).

The "vital and vibrant qualities of nature" (Jordan, 2016) contribute importantly to the therapeutic process out of doors. They also present us with uncertainty; changeable and unpredictable environments that pose challenges to the way we adapt our methods and extend the professional boundaries, which we use to frame our work safely and confidentially with clients. When we work in partnership with nature Berger (2016) suggests that the vitality and ever changing cycles can aid the therapeutic processes of building resilience, developing flexibility and finding a "broader meaning and perspective to difficult stories" (Berger, 2016, p. 179).

Working in nature: health benefits

An emerging evidence-base

Research is beginning to provide us with evidence of the health benefits of being outdoors and engaging with nature in safe and considered activities: "*A body of evidence drawing upon research from environmental psychology has explored the effects of nature upon human perception, emotions, behaviour and cognition*" (Jordan, 2009, p. 28). Kaplan and Kaplan (1989) and Kaplan (1995) established an integrative framework from which to consider the restorative benefits of being in nature. They show how fatigue and stress can be affected positively by walking in natural settings, changing one's environment or gaze, and how entering into a 'compatible environment' reduces cognitive stressors such as problem-solving and directed attention. Richard Louv (2010) presents a compelling case for children to gain more access to nature. He provides evidence of the negative effects on child development, play and behaviour when access is limited or excluded completely. The term nature-decifit-disorder is considered as emerging in parallel with the increased rate of attention-deficit-disorder over the past 40 years.

Berger (2017) argues that "people's estrangement from nature is linked to a broad spectrum of psychosocial disorders and manifestations such as loss of self-esteem and meaning, depression, anxiety, loneliness and alienation" (Berger, 2017, p. 49), and that reconnecting with nature can lead to recovery from trauma, stress and depression. Berger shows how increasing contact with nature and time spent working outdoors increases a stronger body-mind connection, helping people "reach higher levels of consciousness, and widen their spiritual connection and guidance" (Berger, 2017, p. 49). Whilst developing an evidence-base for taking psychotherapy outdoors Jordan (2016) describes how our developmental experiences of nature may have involved using it as a "space for affect regulation and well-being" (Jordan, 2016, p. 66). He shows how working out of doors in nature provides a space for clients to affect-regulate during the therapeutic encounter and how natural, outdoor spaces provide a regulatory space for therapists also, thus enabling them to metabolise difficult emotional material particularly when it is in the form of "projective identification, powerful unconscious material related to abuse and trauma" (Jordan, 2016, p. 66).

Berger (2016, 2017) has developed his approach over many years working in war torn and traumatised communities, combining drama and nature with direct trauma work. Berger and Lahad (2013) describe this work in *The Healing Forest* showing how nature affects how we cope with trauma and how it can help to build resilience. Working with a model which centres on direct creative engagement with nature, they include encouraging remembrance and working with all the senses, imagination, affect and cognition. They have found that movement through these sensory and psychological processes support the client to gain renewed access to resilience and provide a flexibility which endures change thus aiding the recovery from trauma and stress.

Nature also provides a range of naturally occurring energetic experiences that may heighten or enhance health benefits. We perceive these events primarily through our senses as we see, feel, taste, hear and smell our experience of our world. We also move through this experience using these senses, alerting us to changes in temperature, threats in the environment or opening up and feeling ourselves ease into pleasurable sensations. What happens during these physiological movements in the body as our senses react and we experience tension, relaxation, alertness and awe are key to helping us understand how Nature holds and supports our physical and emotional health. The systematic investigation of the physiological effects of

Shinrin-yoku or 'forest bathing' has gathered evidence of the health benefits of 'taking in the forest atmosphere' which includes improved mental and physical relaxation. A major study across 24 forest locations by Park et al. (2010) show that forest environments promote lower concentrations of cortisol, lower pulse rate, lower blood pressure, greater parasympathetic nerve activity and lower sympathetic nerve activity than do city environments.

Li et al. (2008) also showed that forest bathing has a particular affect in relation to our sense of smell. Li's evidence showed that when in a conifer forest, a person breathes in over one hundred different types of phytoncides. These immune boosting vapours released by densely packed coniferous trees were seen to aid stress reduction and gave an increased wellness by lowering inflammation with improved cellular immunity. Exposure to forest soil was also found to increase serotonin levels in the brain. Li et al. provide evidence that our sense of smell absorbs aromatic chemicals that have a significant effect on the limbic system, the part of the brain that regulates memories, emotions and arousal.

The real world: risk and mitigation

The principles of therapeutic practice in the creative arts therapies are guided by a code of ethics defined by each professional association and ratified by a legal and regulatory framework set by the Health and Care Professions Council (HCPC). Whenever we significantly alter the contracted boundary within which therapy takes place we need to ensure, as a primary condition, that these practice standards are maintained at the highest level. The first step we take when considering taking a client out of doors is to seek clarity and advice in relation to our clinical responsibilities and 'duty of care' for the individuals and groups we work with. This will include developing agreed safety protocols, risk assessments and ensure that the work is fully insured. In parallel we will need to assess suitability for this approach in order to maintain clinical efficacy for each individual client.

In terms of ethical practice a central concern is the ability to maintain boundaries and safe containment; for example confidentiality outdoors is fluid, privacy is porous and providing safe psychological spaces in unpredictable environments is problematic. Hasbach (2016) considers the ethical challenges involved when taking clients out of doors and asks whether there is a need for a 'code of ethics' to address the specific issues relating to professional practice. These include "unique concerns as being confidentiality, avoiding harm and professional competence" (Hasbach, 2016, p. 145). The fluidity of the therapeutic boundaries of time, safety, privacy and predictability is examined by Brazier (2016) who maintains that the therapist retains responsibility for the client or group, their "own mental and physical states as well as keeping an awareness of the surrounding terrain and activity in hand" (Brazier, 2016, p. 41). Brazier (2016) has found that the methods and approaches used by therapists working outdoors require an increased awareness of boundary management and assertive responses to infringements from others who may be using the same spaces. Both authors raise concerns around safety and practitioner competence and the need to assess on-going risk when working in different and challenging environments.

In order to work safely and therapeutically Kopytin emphasises how "*eco-arts therapies, like any other therapy, requires appropriately structured and accompanied therapeutic process*" (Kopytin, 2017, p. 39). This position has important implications for the approaches and facilitation methods used. Kopytin places an emphasis on the presence of an active and attentive therapist who is alert, responsive and containing both physically, keeping the space and client safe, and also holding therapeutic process in order to provide the client with "the sense of safety, containment, order and comprehensibility and helps her/him to shape and crystallize experience" (Kopytin, 2017, p. 39). In this respect the therapeutic approach is structured through an active presence holding, supporting and facilitating the client through a creative and therapeutic interaction within nature. The implications for practice are that the therapist will be more active, involved and prepared to co-construct or navigate the therapeutic movement and process in collaboration with the client. This approach will differ from the stance of many conventional therapists and could be a challenge to orthodox practice.

Other ethical issues raised by Whitaker (2016) include how we manage artworks that enter the public domain; the challenges of weather and terrain; changeable and unpredictable environments; and issues relating to access and mobility, comfort and security. She also raises clinical issues relating to the ways in which some individuals may find nature dirty, boring, too risky or too arousing which raises questions around assessment. The fact that the natural world can also evoke, activate or trigger traumatic memory is another important issue which would need to be incorporated into risk assessments on an individual basis.

Risk and benefit assessment

In a clinical context risk assessment and management are essential to making a safe and containing therapeutic space and is an essential part of any therapy process, even more so when the contracted frame is altered radically by moving outside. Hasbach raises the importance of on-going assessment and working within ones professional areas of competency: "it is incumbent on the therapist to assess the level of risk and the client's level of competency and confidence to handle that environment" (Hasbach, 2016, p. 145). Play expert Gill (2007) in *No Fear: Growing Up in a Risk Averse Society* questions the effectiveness of the current philosophy of protecting children from natural environments arguing that childhood is becoming undermined by risk aversion. Gill considers "the role that experience and exposure to risk plays in children's learning and growth" (Gill, 2007, p. 83). In the same way working therapeutically in the outdoors as adults we often access our inner child to explore and understand not only our physical environment but also our emotional and spiritual experience of self. If we eliminate risk completely we constrain our own development and ability to understand ourselves and our limits more fully. What emerges from Gill's work is the need for balanced and robust risk/benefit assessments. These assessments consider the benefits of therapeutic work in the outdoors weighed against the level of risks involved. This approach produces a counter-balance in the risk assessment and is essential when working outdoors in order to allow freedom to explore an outdoor environment safely without removing the inherent challenges.

When assessing risk we find that nature is dynamic and unpredictable (Berger, 2016); it is difficult to predict and tightly manage all risk scenarios and we are challenged as practitioners to maintain safety. In order to hold the work, we are required to keep a wide awareness of what is happening in an ever-changing environment and to provide containment through our presence and boundaried approach (Brazier, 2016). This means that the initial risk assessments relating to the client's needs and abilities, and risks apparent in the location, are not static; they need continual refinement as new and changeable conditions come into the therapy frame and as the client experiences and responds to new challenges.

Conclusion: drawing the threads together

An important aim of this review has been to show how nature-based therapies have been emerging and defining theory and practice through the literature linked to ecopsychology, ecotherapy and psychotherapy (Roszak, 1995; Jordan, 2012). More recently the creative arts therapies have begun to define its unique contributions to theoretical developments which can be shared across disciplines (Kopytin and Rugh, 2017; Atkins and Snyder, 2018). Consequently, what we see in the literature review are examples of arts-based practices and experience which bring something new and innovative to this growing area of professional practice.

Innovation in the area of outdoor therapy groupwork is related to the provision of a safe and structured approach. This has been a repeating theme (Sweeney, 2013; Berger, 2016; Jones et al., 2016). The arts response in all creative arts therapy groupwork requires structure and time: time to arrive, to find or make a space, to create an art response and time to reflect, share and articulate the experience. Sweeney (2013) describes a graduated and focused attention towards a therapeutic interaction in nature, followed by a creative response. Jones et al. (2016) provides a mindfulness walk and art-making structure followed by reflection and making meaning of the experience. Atkins and Snyder (2018) provide a structured and themed groupwork process which leads the group participants through an intentional and creative response within an agreed timeframe.

Working outdoors with individuals also requires structure and accompanied process (Kopytin, 2017). The use of intentional ritual such as an agreed arrival and departure threshold is used to bracket the beginning and ending of a session. More time is required for the journey to, arrival at and return from the session which also needs to be factored in by both therapist and client. Focused and accompanied process is a reoccurring theme described by Brazier (2016) and Hasbach (2016). They stress the importance of the therapist being trained to provide a present, boundaried and active approach when working with individuals and groups out of doors. They also argue that the therapist's role includes facilitating the client's process as well as actively supporting them to find meaning through shared reflective dialogue.

Another theme which emerges is how nature inspires and engages us in multiple ways: sensory, emotionally, cognitively and psychologically. When using the creative therapies outdoors we see a parallel movement into multiple art responses including a visual art response through sculpting, modelling or land art, movement and drama expressed through the body and the use of the voice, sound and rhythm, allowing our experiences to be reflected back at us in nature. The emerging principle described by many practitioners is of being open to an integrative arts approach, in alignment with the expressive arts therapies (McNiff, 2009; Knill et al., 2005).

Environmental arts therapy adds something new to the theoretical developments and practice of the creative arts therapies out of doors. A central factor is the focus upon an indigenous cultural knowledge and reference to the cycle of the turning year. Here in Northern Europe this involves the use of the Celtic Ogham tree calendar as a working model, which provides structured and intentional focus for work with individuals and groups, as well as deepening the practitioner's awareness of the surrounding woodland habitat. There is a greater focus on the seasonal cycles, as referred to by Jordan (2009) and Berger (2016). Environmental arts therapy methods include attuning to the daily, weekly and monthly movement and cycles of the seasons, thus bringing a nuanced attention and attunement to our very personal and intimate relationship within Nature.

References

Atkins, S., and Snyder, M. (2018). *Nature-based expressive arts therapy: Integrating the expressive arts and ecotherapy*. London and Philadelphia, PA: Jessica Kingsley Publishers.

Berger, R. (2009). *Nature therapy: Developing a framework for practice*. PhD thesis, University of Abertay, Dundee, School of Health and Social Sciences.

Berger, R. (2014). Nature therapy: Integrating nature in therapy. In Berger, R. (Ed.), *Arts: The heart of therapy* (pp. 441–443). Kiryat Byalik: Ach Publications.

Berger, R. (2016). Renewed by nature: Nature therapy as a framework to help people deal with crisis, trauma and loss. In Jordan, M., and Hinds, J. (Eds.), *Ecotherapy: Theory, research and practice* (pp. 177–186). London and New York: Palgrave.

Berger, R. (2017). Nature therapy: Highlighting steps for professional development. In Kopytin, A., and Rugh, M. (Eds.), *Environmental expressive therapies: Nature assisted theory and practice*. New York and Oxon: Routledge.

Berger, R., and Lahad, M. (2013). *The healing forest in post-crisis work with children*. London: Jessica Kingsley.

Brazier, C. (2016). Nature-based practice: A Buddhist psychotherapy perspective. In Jordan, M., and Hinds, J. (Eds.), *Ecotherapy: Theory, research and practice* (pp. 32–44). London and New York: Palgrave.

Buzzell, L., and Chalquist, C. (2009). *Ecotherapy: Healing with nature in mind*. San Francisco, CA: Sierra Club Books.

Connell, C. (1998). *Something understood: Art therapy in cancer care*. London: Wrexham Publications.

Davies, J. (1999). Environmental art therapy: Metaphors in the field. *The Arts in Psychotherapy*, 26 (4), pp. 45–49.

Davies, J. (2017). Drawing nature. In Kopytin, A., and Rugh, M. (Eds.), *Environmental expressive therapies: Nature assisted theory and practice* (pp. 63–77). New York and Oxon: Routledge.

Dodds, J. (2012). The ecology of phantasy: Ecopsychoanalysis and the three ecologies. In Rust, M.J., and Totton, N. (Eds.), *Vital signs: Psychological responses to ecological crisis* (pp. 119–132). London: Karnac Books.

Gifford, J. (2000). *The Celtic wisdom of trees: Mysteries, magic and medicine*. Alresford, Hants, UK: Godsfield Press Ltd.

Gill, T. (2007). *No fear: Growing up in a risk averse society*. London: Calouste Gulbenkian Foundation.

Graves, R. (1948). *The white goddess: A historical grammar of poetic myth*. London: Faber & Faber.

Guattari, F. (2000). *The three ecologies*. London: Continuum.

Hageneder, F. (2000). *The spirit of trees: Science, symbiosis and inspiration*. Edinburgh: Floris Books.

Hageneder, F. (2001). *The heritage of trees: History, culture and symbolism*. Edinburgh: Floris Books.

Hasbach, P. (2016). Prescribing nature: Techniques, challenges and ethical considerations. In Jordan, M., and Hinds, J. (Eds.), *Ecotherapy: Theory, research and practice* (pp. 138–147). London and New York: Palgrave.

Jones, V., Thompson, B., and Watson, J. (2016). Feet on the ground and branching out: Being with nature as a tool for recovery in crisis within NHS mental health services. In Jordan, M., and Hinds, J. (Eds.), *Ecotherapy: Theory, research and practice* (pp. 162–176). London and New York: Palgrave.

Jordan, M. (2009). Back to nature. *Therapy Today*, April, pp 28–30.

Jordan, M. (2012). Did Lacan go camping? Psychotherapy in search of an ecological self. In Rust, M.J., and Totton, N. (Eds.), *Vital signs: Psychological responses to ecological crisis* (pp. 133–145). London: Karnac Books.

Jordan, M., and Hinds, J. (2016). *Ecotherapy: Theory, research and practice*. London and New York: Palgrave.

Kalmanowitz, D., and Lloyd, B. (1997). *The Portable Studio: Art therapy and political conflict: Initiatives in the former Yugoslavia and KwaZulu-Natal, South Africa*. London: Health Education Authority.

Kalmanowitz, D., and Lloyd, B. (2005). *Art therapy and political violence: With art, without illusion*. London and New York: Routledge.

Kaplan, H. (2019). *You as a tree*. Blurb.co.uk online publishing.

Kaplan, R., and Kaplan, S. (1989). *The experience of nature: A psychological perspective*. Cambridge MA: Cambridge University Press.

Kaplan, S. (1995). The restorative benefits of nature: Towards an integrative framework. *Journal of Environmental Psychology*, 15, pp. 169–182.

Knill, P.J., Levine, E.G., and Levine, S.K. (2005). *Principles and practice of expressive arts therapy: Towards a therapeutic aesthetics*. London and Philadelphia, PA: Jessica Kingsley Publisher.

Kopytin, A. (2016). Green studio: Eco-perspective on the therapeutic setting in art therapy. In Kopytin, A., and Rugh, M. (Eds.), *The Green studio: Nature and arts in therapy* (pp. 3–26). New York: Nova Science.

Kopytin, A. (2017). Environmental and ecological expressive therapies: The emerging conceptual framework for practice. In Kopytin, A., and Rugh, M. (Eds.), *Environmental expressive therapies: Nature assisted theory and practice* (pp. 23–47). New York and Oxon: Routledge.

Kopytin, A., and Rugh, M. (2016). *The Green studio: Nature and arts in therapy*. New York: Nova Science.

Kopytin, A., and Rugh, M. (2017). *Environmental expressive therapies: Nature assisted theory and practice*. New York and Oxon: Routledge.

Li, Q., Morimoto, K., Kobayashi, M., Inagaki, H., Katsumata, M., and Hirata, Y. (2008). Visiting a forest, but not a city, increases human natural killer activity and expression of anti-cancer proteins. *International Journal of Immunopathological Pharmacology*, 21 (1), pp. 117–127.

Louv, R. (2010). *Last child in the woods: Saving our children from Nature-deficit disorder*. Croydon: CPI Group.

McNiff, S. (1992). *Art as medicine: Creating a therapy of the imagination*. Boston: Shambhala Publications.

McNiff, S. (2009) *Integrating the arts in therapy: History, theory and practice*. Springfield, IL: Charles Thomas Publisher.

McNiff, S. (2016). Pandora's gifts: Using imagination and all of the arts in therapy. In Rubin, J. (Ed.), *Approaches to art therapy: Theory and technique* (3rd edition, pp. 468–478). New York and London: Routledge.

Milner, M. (1957). *On not being able to paint*. London: Heinemann Educational Books Ltd.

Park, B.J., Tsunetsugu, Y., Kagawa, T., and Miyazaki, Y. (2010). The physiological effects of Shinrin-yoku (taking in the forest atmosphere or forest bathing): Evidence from field experiments in 24 forests across Japan. *Environmental Health and Preventive Medicine*, 15 (1), pp. 18–26.

Patterson, J.M. (1996). *Tree wisdom: The definitive guidebook to the myth, folklore and healing power of trees*. London and San Francisco, CA: Harper Collins Publishers.

Pfeifer, E. (2017). Music-nature-therapy: Outdoor music therapy and other nature-related approaches in music therapy. In Kopytin, A., and Rugh, M. (Eds.), *Environmental expressive therapies: Nature assisted theory and practice* (pp. 177–203). New York and Oxon: Routledge.

Roszak, T. (1992). *The voice of the earth: An exploration of ecopsychology*. London: Simon and Schuster.

Roszak, T. (1995). Where psyche meets Gaia. In Roszak, T., Gomes, M., and Kanner, A.D. (Eds.), *Ecopsychology: Restoring the earth, healing the mind* (pp. 1–17). San Francisco, CA: Sierra Club Books.

Roszak, T. (2009). A psyche as big as the earth. In Buzzell, L., and Chalquist, C. (Eds.), *Ecotherapy: Healing with nature in mind* (pp. 30–36). San Francisco, CA: Sierra Club Books.

Rust, M.J. (2012). Ecological intimacy. In Rust, M.J., and Totton, N. (Eds.), *Vital signs: Psychological responses to ecological crisis* (pp. 149–161). London: Karnac Books.

Rust, M.J., and Totton, N. (2012). *Vital signs: Psychological responses to ecological crisis*. London: Karnac Books.

Schaverien, J. (1989). The picture within the frame. In Gilroy, A., and Dalley, T. (Eds.), *Pictures at an exhibition* (pp. 147–155). London and New York: Routledge.

Siddons Heginworth, I. (2008). *Environmental arts therapy and the tree of life*. Exeter: Spirits Rest Books.

Siddons Heginworth, I., Kaplan, H., and Nash, G. (2013). *Environmental arts therapy course handbook*. London: London Art Therapy Centre.

Sweeney, T. (2013). *Eco-art therapy: Creativity that let the Earth Teach*. ISBN 0-6159-0147-6.

Totton, N. (2011). *Wild therapy: Undomesticating inner and outer worlds*. Ross-on-Wye: PCCS Books.

Totton, N. (2012). Nothings out of order: Towards an ecological therapy. In Rust, M.J., and Totton, N. (Eds.), *Vital signs: Psychological responses to ecological crisis* (pp. 253–264). London: Karnac Books.

Whitaker, P. (2016). Review of the Green Studio: Nature and the arts in therapy. *American Journal of Art Therapy*, 33 (4), pp. 220–221.

PART II

Childhood, love and attachment

The heart of the matter

3

THE WILD INSIDE

Offering children natural materials and an ecopsychological understanding of self within art therapy

Lydia Boon

Introduction

Since completing my training as an art psychotherapist, I have worked with children and adolescents attending schools within Bristol including one within a particularly disadvantaged catchment area, and therefore I work with some of our most vulnerable yet inspiring and courageous children. It has not yet been possible for me to practice environmental arts therapy outdoors with these students, so instead I bring an array of natural materials and objects into the art therapy room. This depends on what I find seasonally and generally includes sand, clay, earth, stones, shells, leaves, sticks, charcoal and feathers. These can simply be explored or touched, used as or with art materials, or they might inspire ideas for creative play, imagination and discussion within therapy. My motivation for doing this was a result of my own experiences in nature and using natural materials in my own creative process. I have found this profoundly moving, nurturing and reassuring at times when life has been at its most challenging, both recently as an adult, but also at times in my childhood. There I found something more than just what the people around me could offer. I came to believe that a greater awareness of our complex interrelatedness with nature and knowledge of natural cycles, biological and material processes and getting 'in touch' with the qualities of natural substances can help to provide context and grounding for emotional, psychological and environmental challenges. Since introducing natural materials into art therapy, I have found that children gravitate towards the natural objects with curiosity and interest which seems to catalyse imaginative and meaningful expression. Drawing from ecopsychology, neuroscience and child developmental theory, I have sought to understand the benefits that seem evident when offering environmental arts therapy to children, even when sessions are conducted indoors. I include three vignettes taken from my work with children, as observations within art therapy laid the ground for the concepts explored here (permissions have been given and the identity of the individuals hidden to protect confidentiality).

More than human

Bringing nature into the art therapy room and expanding the concept of the 'self' to include an 'ecological self' might well offer children something integral and sorely needed in these particularly complex and challenging times. Jung and Franz (1964) identified that in Western culture there is an over valuing of the rational, factual, reductionist and scientific disciplines and less value given to the creative, instinctual, experiential and feeling based disciplines. This I believe is reflected within the current pedagogical mainstream. Despite well-meaning teachers, the school system leaves little opportunity for self-directed, creative or exploratory learning and children are under ever more pressure to reach target grades and pass exams. They are continuously compared to each other in ability, effort and intelligence. Even the way the creative arts are delivered often leaves little room for improvisation or creative self-expression. Synonymous with this, children have limited opportunity to develop their own sense of deeper meaning, purpose or spirituality beyond what they may be exposed to within their family (Jackson, 2016).

The educational system reflects a modern-day position that puts us as spectators, distinguishable and distant from the natural world, seeing it as something 'out there', a resource, something to fear, manage or protect. The Cartesian mind-body split parallels a self-Nature split. This dis-connect moves us away from ways of knowing only found in relation to our more-than-human nature. To some degree we have lost touch with our inner compass, a moral tether and spiritual connection that transcend culture.

> Modern Man does not understand how much his 'rationalism' has put him at odds with the underworld. Freed from superstition (so he believes), but has also lost spiritual values to a dangerous degree. His moral spiritual tradition has disintegrated and he is now paying the price for this break up in world disorientation and dissociation.
>
> *(Jung and Franz, 1964, p. 94)*

This price is becoming evident both individually and globally (Roszak et al., 1995). Destruction of ecosystems that fundamentally support life is a real and serious threat to humanity today and more so for future generations. Whether they are fully aware of this or not, our youth are growing up facing huge uncertainty about the sustainability and stability of their world unparalleled in human history. It is likely that the undercurrents of this growing collective awareness, or the denial and dissociation from it, is adding to anxiety and dis-ease amongst them. Simultaneously children are spending less time in direct contact with Nature and so experiencing less opportunity for meaningful and treasured experiences there that would cultivate a sense of relatedness and attachment to the non-human world

(Lee, 2012). Aside from the alarming global cost there are growing research studies that show the negative impacts upon children deprived of contact with nature. Louv (2005) used the term 'nature deficit disorder' to describe the direct human cost of alienation from the natural world including diminished use of the senses, attention difficulties and higher rates of physical and emotional illness. There is a growing body of research showing the negative impacts upon children deprived of contact with nature (Annerstedt and Währborg, 2011) and conversely many studies that show, "what is gained biologically, cognitively and spiritually, through positive physical connection to Nature" (Louv, 2005, p. 34).

It is evident through my work with children and teenagers that the world is ever more complex and challenging for them. Children's mental health issues continue to grow, as statistics show at least 1 in 10 children have a diagnosable mental health disorder; that is roughly three children in every classroom (Green, 2005). The Office for National Statistics Online (2015) found that suicide was the most common cause of death for both boys (17% of all deaths) and girls (11%) aged between 5 and 19.

Children are generally spending significantly less time interacting face to face with adults, each other and less time in contact with the natural world. Instead they are spending increasing amounts of time in front of screens with information and a one-dimensional stimulation constantly fed to them through online worlds of gaming, chat and media. As Louv points out, "it's not that screens and technology are detrimental per say, but what children are missing when they are using them" (Louv, 2005, p. 136). The intense, often relentless hyper-connectivity that social media creates with an ever-pressing search for recognition, acceptance or to be 'liked', paradoxically leads to a definite growing sense of insecurity and social anxiety amongst children who are spending large amounts of time online. Their online interactions reflect a primal basic human need for acceptance; however, any reassurance in this regard seems short-lived. 'Likes' appear to be undermined by the superficiality and untruthfulness of 'online persona', creating a growing chasm between authenticity and acceptability.

Barrows (1995) draws our attention to the fact that established psychological theories, including all developmental psychology, have neglected to consider the importance of the role of the natural world within human development and mental health. Hillman and Ventura echo this, "psychotherapy has not gone far enough in its thinking, that by focusing on the internal makeup or the family of origin of the client, it has not connected to the wider world and is therefore incapable of treating the individual" (Hillman and Ventura, 1992, p. 54). Evidence from neuroscience and psychology support this idea by showing that a child's psyche is part of a vast synergistic model of connections reaching beyond human interaction (Feral, 1998). McNiff (2004), followed by Kopytin and Rugh (2017), voice concerns that even within art therapy we often limit ourselves to the assumptions of these mainstream psychological constructs. They suggest a new vision in which the art material or object which is being used by the child is instead related to as a subject in its own right. This less anthropocentric view facilitates awareness of the object or material as having a history, a narrative, and takes into account its particular physical qualities to acknowledge the 'life' of the subject. For example, a stick was once part of a tree, it had nutrients from the ground, warmth and light from the sun, rain in order to grow from a seed or nut into tree. It may have lost branches in a storm or have been hit by lightning; it may be reaching branches up to the sky in glory or slumped over like an old man. Any of these observations regarding its physical quality and position in the world and its relationship to other elements and creatures can lead a child to their own experiences. In this and other ways environmental arts therapy utilises nature as 'co-therapist' (Jordan, 2014), which further democratises the space of therapy (Berger, 2006). This allows for 'psychic space' from conscious or unconscious agendas within schools, families or wider society; allowing both therapist and client to find different and new ways of relating, freeing up ways of thinking about the issues and problems (Jordan, 2014).

Objectives set with a 'means to an end' and goal-orientated activities have their place in helping children to learn all manner of important life and academic skills; however, overemphasis on them may leave a child out of touch with their own inner wellspring of natural curiosity. Nature allows for undirected learning and a way of being that is not goal orientated but seeks self-motivation and self-oriented meaning. Hilgers (1997) went so far as to say that when children have a strong conception of relatedness to the earth, there is likely to be a stronger sense of bonding with the self. Roszak et al. (1995) and others have called this an 'ecological self'. The 'natural mind' Jung said, "*springs from natural sources, and not from opinions taken from books; it wells up from the earth like a natural spring, and brings with it the peculiar wisdom of nature*" (Jung, 1963, p. 50).

Nature mask

Tania, a thirteen-year-old girl of Afro-Caribbean descent, came to me for art therapy sessions within a school situated in a predominantly white area of the city where there are pervasive issues of violence, drug abuse and anti-social behaviour within the community. Tania described incidents of racial abuse from children at school and from those in her local community that had left her feeling considerably unsafe and untrusting of others. She was struggling with friendships, becoming isolated, and finding it hard to differentiate between general insensitivity or rudeness at school, or the possibility that she was being treated differently because of her race. Tania felt other's expectations acutely and had become very anxious about doing 'well enough' at school. She had begun to question her own self-worth and she told me she felt she was losing herself.

Tania chose to use clay and to make a mask (Figure 3.1). This was something that she thought of after seeing a template mask on the shelf. As she held the clay and shaped it, she told me about waking up early, watching the sunrise over the city before she left for school, how the beauty of it gave her a sense of calm and reassurance. As she rolled the clay out, she reflected on places and times she had felt free to be herself, less anxious and more hopeful. She remembered when her family, years ago, had driven to Scotland and she had looked out at the mountains and

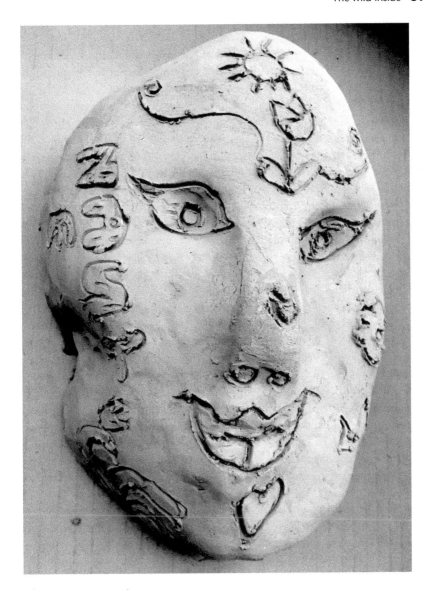

FIGURE 3.1   Nature mask

felt amazed by them. She concluded that she felt free to be herself when outside in nature. The clay mask took shape and she told me as she drew 'owl eyes', mountains, the sun, waves, a flower and a heart, "this is my nature mask, it's peaceful, it sees beauty and doesn't judge". For Tania this mask, intentionally left as raw clay became an important reminder of the peace and acceptance that she felt in herself when in nature and helped her find stability from which to explore the turbulent social world around her.

I feel therefore I am

Within the profession of art therapy we need to gain a deeper intrinsic and clinical understanding of the qualities of the materials that we offer to clients and their responses to them (Snir and Regev, 2013; Sholt and Gavron, 2006). In the light of research, reading other's work and my own work with children and teenagers, it seems to me that natural materials are particularly engaging for them. They reach out to explore them, and seem naturally excited by them (Courtney, 2017; White, 2004). It is possible that our evolutionary relationship with nature and our neurological development over this time is in part responsible for this. We have a 'biophilic' locus (Wilson, 1986) that has enabled us to survive and thrive. Until relatively very recent history it was imperative for survival that we achieve an intimate understanding and awareness of nature, its materials, organisms, processes and cycles; many argue that it still is. Contact with nature has been a fundamental and inseparable part of the development of our physical, behavioural, social and psychological evolution, from life as single celled organisms to our position as Homo sapiens. Lee puts it: "our children have been right at the centre of all this, spontaneously, routinely, and unavoidably participating in sustained, close, and progressive interaction with animals and their habitats" (Lee, 2012, p. 194). Nature remains an incredibly important teacher for us despite modern-day living, which creates an illusion of independence and security from nature's wild places and the challenges therein.

With neuroimagery we now know that the brain is only a third of its full size at birth and develops through infancy and childhood in much the same order that the brain developed over the history of our evolution (Perry, 2006). This begins with the primitive central nervous system, the 'reptilian brain', and then grows outwards to incorporate brain regions which enable the development of attributes considered more human, such as the ability to plan, self-regulate, control impulses, problem-solve, imagine and form symbols and therefore language (Panksepp and Biven, 2012).

Gordon Orians, professor of zoology at Washington University, puts it succinctly as: "we have evolutionary remnants of past experiences hard-wired into a species nervous system" (cited in Louv, 2005, p. 47). Many in the field of psychology – in particular those working with children with any developmental issues who have experienced abuse, neglect or early relational trauma, now recognise that a successful treatment need take into account the psycho-biological mechanisms between infant, their surroundings and their primary caregiver. Schore acknowledges a paradigm shift from the dominance of behavioural and cognitive psychology to a focus on 'bodily based emotions' and 'psychobiological states' (Schore, 2010, p. 4) that no longer negate the importance of "ancient emotional systems that have a power that is quite independent from neocortical cognitive processes" (Panksepp and Biven, 2012, p. 51). Children who have had early adverse experiences require therapeutic intervention that includes engagement at the level of bodily based sensory-emotional activity including touch, sound, image and movement that stimulates the senses and also allow for regulation (Levine, 2010).

It is this stimulation and also regulation of the autonomic nervous system (ANS) that takes place within therapy which enables the process in which information moves from one area of the brain to another. Fragmented somatic experiences held in the body's unconscious memory, creating implicit trauma-related expectations, continue to trigger stress responses (fight/flight/freeze/flop) in the amygdala (Rothschild, 2000). In accessing these and regulating stress response information can be processed and moved to the hippocampus, where it can be understood in context and stored autobiographically. Contextualisation and understanding of emotionally intense experiences is only possible in attunement with another mind (in infancy this would be the mind of the parent or within therapy, that of the therapist) and through a process of 'mentalisation', the capacity "to feel, whilst thinking about feeling" (Fonagy, 2001). This requires presence and mindfulness of the therapist/caregiver; however, the quality and sensory nature of the environment may well influence this process significantly also. We now know that experiences in nature both stimulate and regulate the ANS. Contact with natural objects, which children so readily seek out and touch, seem to reconnect them with their bodily senses and emotional responses whilst also creating calm. Nature's plethora of sensory information, an 'infinite reservoir' (Louv, 2005, p. 65) allows them chances to link the exterior world with the interior hidden affective world. Natural forms and materials within art therapy invite children to use their hands and engage in playful, healthy touch. This is perhaps more so than when using artificial art materials, which generally seem less nuanced, more simplistic in form and texture and do not always invite explorative touch.

Experiences of healthy touch create "mild sedation, decreases in blood pressure and aids in autonomic nervous system regulation and cardiovascular health" (Cozolino, 2006, p. 103; Weller and Feldman, 2003). Rothschild adds that "increasing sense of boundary at the skin level will often reduce hyper-arousal and increase the feeling of control over one's own body" (Rothschild, 2000, p. 146). Natural forms seem particularly useful for developing haptic/touch perception as they are likely to 'tap into' evolutionary hard wiring and due to this increase the likelihood of a shift in 'primary process affective states' (Panksepp and Biven, 2012). Elbrecht and Antcliff explain that, [as] "patients learn to tolerate being aware of their physical experiences, they discover physical impulses and options that they had abandoned for the sake of survival during trauma" (Elbrecht and Antcliff, 2014, p. 24). Manipulating substances such as clay, sand and other natural materials offer a necessary and direct experience of potency and control (Henley, 2002; Elbrecht, 2013).

Our sensory worlds have been dramatically dulled down compared to what we would have experienced over the main course of human evolution. This means a dramatic reduction in bodily sensory awareness, which may also affect emotional regulation systems and emotional resilience. Jung warned that "in the civilising process, we have increasingly divided our consciousness from the deeper instinctive strata of the human psyche, and even ultimately from the somatic basic of psychic phenomenon" (cited in Sabini, 2002, p. 93). Louv (2005) also warns of this modern high-tech, dulled-down environment and its propensity to produce children with a 'know-it-all' attitude. Yet he also reminds us that this mind set is "fragile and in a flash it can burn and give way to something essential that emerges in its ashes" (Louv, 2005, p. 69).

Wild Amazonian man

Esther was eight years old and referred to me by concerned teachers who described her as disruptive, disaffected, rude to staff and unkind to other children. She presented a 'know-it-all' and 'I don't care' attitude and clearly a protective front. It was Esther's first art therapy session and I let her know that she could choose what she wanted to play with or make. Esther spotted a tray of natural materials next to a large bag of clay, looked at me and asked, "can I use those as well?" She began looking closely at the objects inside the tray, taking out a seed pod to examine. Then with my help she grabbed handfuls of clay energetically. "I'm not going to tell you what I'm making, you have to guess."

"Ok". I said, and I watched her press, shape and bash the clay for several minutes until she had a ball. Twigs became arms, a beech nut shell for a nose, a red berry and a small pine cone as eyes and a large scraggly mossy beard. She looked at me and asked "can you see what it is?" I said it looked to me like it might be a person. She gave me a wry smile and said "yes but what kind of person?" I did not know so she told me: "he's a wild man from the Amazon". I wondered aloud how he might be feeling here, away from the rainforest where he lived. She replied without hesitation "he feels nervous and worried that he doesn't have any friends, but also kind of excited, because it's all new and different". I asked her if there is anything she would like to make or give him that might help him feel calmer or reassured. She said she would make him a headdress, and set about finding feathers, twigs ferns and leaves. The wild man with his headdress seemed elevated to a tribal chief and I enquired as to whether he felt differently now. Esther said, "he feels proud and important, more special". There were evident parallels between Esther's experiences at home and school and I said that even though we are all special and important, we don't always feel that way. She nodded thoughtfully.

It was raining outside and as the session had progressed the sky had grown darker. At that moment we both noticed a flash, our eyes meeting in a moment of surprise; then I saw her awe and excitement. It was lightning, shortly followed by the deep roll of thunder. She rushed to the window and we stood side by side looking out and up into the blanket of cloud expectantly. "I love lightening", she said, "I'm not like others in my class, I don't like computers, I'd much rather be outside. I hate school. I want to be a tribal person in the Amazon". I felt that she was sharing with me the pain of not belonging, of not feeling accepted at school amongst her peers and perhaps not feeling good enough there. The sky flashed again. I asked her if lightning led her to imagine anything. "Frankenstein" she replied, "but I find it exciting not scary". Deep rumbles added impact to the mental image. In this first session Esther was drawn to, physically engaged with and inspired by the natural materials and the lightening phenomenon. These had allowed her to approach some difficult feelings at a safe distance, created a rich source of material for our work together, as well as offering opportunity to connect in awe and fascination at nature, enabling a positive first step in developing a positive relationship between us.

Nature inspires imagination

It may be nature's qualities that engage the sensory emotional systems of children and speak to their archetypal experiences that so ignites their imagination. This is reflected in studies that show children's imaginative play increases in nature (Courtney, 2017; White, 2004). Nicholson (1971) refers to natural objects as 'loose parts' and attributes some of their tendency to stimulate imagination to the fact that they can be transformed and used in infinite ways. They offer substance, form, colour, texture, and a narrative, whilst allowing enough freedom for a child to engage imaginatively and transform the object into something completely different. Santostefano stated that "Nature has power to shape the psyche and play a significant role in helping traumatised children" (1999 cited in Louv, 2005, p. 51). By allowing projections and by offering more freedom than toys that already have meaning attached, "you're giving the child the opportunity to express what is within" (Santostefano, 1999 cited in Louv, 2005, p. 51). Traditional art materials, indeed any expressive medium, can allow for creative expression; however, some individuals, even at primary school age, can find the blank page intimidating. Imagined expectations can block expression, making a 'way in' hard to find. Unfortunately, even young children have often already been influenced by limiting concepts around creativity and adopt a feeling of not being 'good enough' at art. Natural materials seem to offer a bypass to this block and free some children up to enjoy a more playful and imaginative creative expression. Nature's metaphors flourish. By offering shape, form, colour, texture and narrative, nature provides contact with emotional material surrounding archetypal human experiences, often arising in relation to significant life events such as birth, death, loss and transition. However, it does so at a safe enough distance, so as not to overwhelm, allowing these aspects to be grappled with instead of being pushed into the shadows.

Guns, bridges and portals

When I first met Justin for art therapy sessions, he was nine. He was preoccupied and burdened, and he was finding life hard at home and at school. The adults around him expressed confusion and despair about him as he was clearly bright but always on the defensive and had frequent angry outbursts. Within therapy he seemed keen for me to like him and to think of him as 'good', however he kept his feelings at bay, presenting himself as calm and rational as he spoke about arguments at home and accusations that others had made about him. Justin was not drawn to using art materials for the first few weeks and despite talking a lot, I felt that he was resisting moving into his emotions. It was during the seventh session with Justin that he chose to use natural materials. He looked surprised as he hadn't noticed the box containing them before and asked me what they were for. I said that they were there to look at, to touch, to inspire imagination and stories or to use to make things, whatever he would like. He took out several objects, stroking soft feathers against the back of his hand, carefully minding the spikes whilst forcing open a hardened chestnut shell and then picking up a thick stick that had a curve like a handle. He said, "it's like a gun".

"Oh, yes I see", I said, acknowledging his interpretation, possibly a symbolic representation of his anger, fear, or the need for protection. Justin became absorbed in painting the stick/gun and then he stuck it upright into a ball of clay and returned to the box of natural materials to find another stick, adding it to the first to make what looked like a bridge. He seemed to be allowing himself to move into a creative process. Frustration arose when his structure collapsed. I felt acutely his need to make it work as he secured it with more clay adding moss and paint until he looked up towards me at its completion. He said, "it's weird, but cool, like a bridge, or a passage". "Ah yes I can see that", I replied, "if it's a passage I wonder what is on the other side?"

Clearly now a little proud of his creation, Justin said "well it's a portal, I guess, to another world". I asked him what we might see if we went through. Justin said if he could go anywhere it would be back in time. "I'd go back to see granddad". He became quiet, head down and tears came. Following this we spoke about his grandfather who had passed away just over a year ago and had been the only person who Justin felt had loved him no matter what. He'd been there for him throughout his mum and dad's divorce. Given space to be with these feelings, I then pointed out what a powerful and important image he had created. Justin could see the link between his anger, his tears of sadness and his grief. He felt he had no one he could talk to. He said that his father never gets upset, only angry. For his father being strong meant hiding sadness, hurt and even affection. He was reluctant to share his feelings with his mother, as he felt abandoned by her because she had started a relationship with another man who in Justin's experience was strict and unkind. The natural materials seemed to allow Justin a 'way in' to a creative imaginative process and in doing so led him to his feelings.

Connection and belonging

Since Bowlby's research conducted in the 1960s, it has been accepted that early infant-caregiver experiences influence the quality of attachment within the first few years of life and lay the foundations for future relationships and impact a child's development right into adulthood, even affecting their future offspring. Now we understand in far greater detail the significant qualities of these formative relationships. Schore describes 'Optimal attachment communications' between infant and caregiver that achieve 'neuro-biological synchronisation', which "affects the maturation of brain regions that processes and regulate somatic aspects of emotion" (Schore, 2010, p. 28).

Experiences of nature may well significantly impact the child-parent dyad within these first few years. Trevarthen (1993) terms the attachment forming interactions between infant-caregiver as 'primary intersubjectivity'. Just as important in this process of connection between parent and infant are the spaces between connection, in which the infant looks away to regulate and 'digest' intense affect neurochemicals (Stern, 2002). The infant begins to experience herself as a separate autonomous being. Simultaneously she is connecting and becoming 'one' with her surroundings. Barrows (1995) reminds us that the infant has awareness not only of human touch but of the breeze on their skin, variations in light, colour, temperature, texture and sound. Shepard (1998) goes so far as to say that the environmental context of the infant-mother relationship is a 'second grounding', the environment is something to be swallowed, internalised and incorporated as the self. The more their spontaneous gestures in response to stimuli are in turn responded to as meaningful, the more children experience themselves as intentional beings, and eventually understand more fully the meanings their own actions carry.

Then at approximately nine months, shared experiences of sensory-emotional responses to nature are also likely to be important when 'secondary intersubjectivity' occurs (Trevarthen, 1993). The infant becomes aware of her mother as a separate thinking and feeling entity and becomes interested in her responses to the world around them, to begin to imagine and make sense of what she may be feeling and thinking. A dulled down sensory environment may make this process much less available to the developing infant. Given that "*even brief experiences of mutual recognition and shared dyadic consciousness strengthen the relationship*" (Van Der Heide, 2012, p. 41), nature may play a fundamental role in secure attachment by offering greater opportunity for connection and 'joint attention'.

In addition to this, nature provides a container or a 'scapegoat' and a safe way to experience interpersonal connection, protecting the relationship when relating directly feels too threatening. This allows the therapist and child to stand side by side, the difficulty being 'out there' until experiences can be owned. Research by Wells (cited in Louv, 2005) found that anxiety, depression, and behavioural misconduct were lower for those living in high nature environments, perhaps due to the green spaces providing better opportunity for socialising and shared experiences.

In some ways, natural materials, especially clay and sand due to their malleability, can offer a subtly responsive and reflective relationship allowing children to experience 'me–not me'. Instead of relating directly to another being, which can be intolerable in cases of early relational trauma, they can begin to relate to the projections within the form (Jordan, 2014). This provides the therapist with greater information about the internal world of the child and an opportunity to relate to the object and so 'reach' the child there. Natural materials can also allow for safe expression of aggression (Sholt and Gavron, 2006; Henley, 2002). Breaking a stick is not the same as breaking a paintbrush or a pencil. It gives licence and a container for healthy expression of anger not directed at themselves, the therapist or the room. The sense of potency and control that comes with this, such as in the creation of mess and the symbolic expressions of defense, is a necessary part of moving through anger to fear and grief beneath. It offers children a way to these feelings and importantly a way through them. The joyful and positive experiences that children generally find in nature and with natural objects seem to provide a safe place and a base to return to when difficult feelings would otherwise be overwhelming.

Summary

As art therapists we can utilise nature as 'co-therapist' to safely approach existential themes of life, death, change, renewal, loss and new beginnings. Nature's endless cycles teach us to embrace and to let go, to nurture and be nurtured, to find strength and to accept our limits. For children this can be invaluable as learning about the absolutes in nature, that can't be changed, rationalised away or argued with, provides boundaries and limits that are deeply humbling and remind us of our shared human condition. Here we can all relate regardless of age, gender or race. Learning the limits of human knowledge allows us to relinquish responsibility for those things outside our control. Nature becomes the ultimate rule setter, nurturer and teacher, a superior parent (Kopytin and Rugh, 2017) which for all children is important especially for those who have not had good enough parenting. The experience of nature presents children with something so much greater than they are, an environment where they can grapple with concepts of infinity and eternity and experience the elements and natural cycles, as Louv says: "without which we forget our place; we forget that larger fabric on which our lives depend" (Louv, 2005, p. 97).

A relationship with nature, I believe, is of crucial importance, given our contemporary society with its ever-seductive ways for our children to disconnect, dull their senses and disappear into cyber realities at their detriment; when cultivated within art therapy it is a relationship that might last a lifetime and remain beneficial far beyond the end of therapy. It is a relationship that invites new (old) ways of relating to self, others and the world around, one that is grounded in sensory, emotional and imaginative shared experiences.

References

Annerstedt, M., and Währborg, P. (2011). Nature-assisted therapy: Systematic review of controlled and observational studies. *Scandinavian Journal of Public Health*, 39, pp. 371–388.

Barrows, A. (1995). The ecopsychology of development. In Roszak, T., Gomes, M.E., and Kanner, A.D. (eds.), *Ecopsychology: Restoring the earth, healing the mind.* San Francisco, CA: Sierra Club Books.

Berger, R. (2006). Using contact with nature, creativity and rituals as a therapeutic medium with children with learning difficulties: A case study. *Emotional & Behavioural Difficulties*, 11 (2), pp. 135–147.

Courtney, J.A. (2017). The art of utilizing the metaphorical elements of Nature as "co-therapist' in ecopsychology play therapy (pp. 100–122). In Kopytin, A., and Rugh, M. (Eds.), *Environmental expressive therapies: Nature assisted theory and practice.* New York: Routledge.

Cozolino, L. (2006). *The neuroscience of human relationships.* New York: W.W. Norton & Company.

Elbrecht, C. (2013). *Trauma healing at the clay field: A sensorimotor art therapy approach.* London: Jessica Kingsley Publishers.

Elbrecht, C., and Antcliff, L.R. (2014). Being touched through touch. Trauma treatment through haptic perception at the Clay Field: A sensorimotor art therapy. *International Journal of Art Therapy*, 19 (1), pp. 19–30.

Feral, C-H. (1998). Healing practices in ecopsychology: The connectedness model and optimal development: Is ecopsychology the answer to emotional well-being? *Journal of Humanistic Psychology and Ecopsychology*, 26 (1–3), pp. 243–274. Published online: 16 August 2010.

Fonagy, P. (2001). *Attachment theory and psychoanalysis.* London: Karnac.

Green, H. (2005). *Mental health of children & young people in Great Britain.* Basingstoke: Palgrave.

Henley, D. (2002). *Clayworks in art therapy: Plying the sacred circle.* London: Jessica Kingsley Publishers.

Hilgers, L. (1997). Earth-friendly therapy. *Self*, 19, p. 70.

Hillman, J., and Ventura, M. (1992). *We've had hundreds of years of psychotherapy and the world's getting worse.* San Francisco, CA: HarperCollins.

Jackson, U. (2016). *Girls rising: A guide to nurturing a confident and soulful adolescent.* Berkeley, CA: Parallax Press.

Jordan, M. (2014). Moving beyond counselling and psychotherapy as it currently is – taking therapy outside. *European Journal of Psychotherapy & Counselling*, 16 (4), pp. 361–375.

Jung, C.G. (1963). *Memories, dreams, reflections.* New York, NY: Crown Publishing Group/ Random House.

Jung, C.G., and Franz, M.L. (1964). *Man and his symbols.* New York: Dell Pub. Co.

Kopytin, A., and Rugh, M. (2017). *Environmental expressive therapies: Nature assisted theory and practice.* New York: Routledge.

Lee, P.C. (2012). The human child's nature orientation. *Child Development Perspectives*, 6 (2), pp. 193–198.

Levine, P.A. (2010). *In an unspoken voice: How the body releases trauma and restores goodness.* Berkeley, CA: North Atlantic Books.

Louv, R. (2005). *Last child in the woods: Saving our children from nature-deficit disorder.* Chapel Hill, NC: Algonquin Books.

McNiff, S. (2004). *Art heals: How creativity cures the soul.* Boston: Shambhala Publications.

Nicholson, S. (1971). How not to cheat children: Theory of loose parts. *Landscape Architecture*, 62 (1), pp. 30–40.

Office for National Statistics Online. (2015). Retrieved from: www.ons.gov.uk/people populationandcommunity/birthsdeathsandmarriages/deaths/bulletins/deathsregistered inenglandandwalesseriesdr/2015#number-of-land-transport-accidents-among-5-to-19-year-olds-decreases.

Panksepp, J., & Biven, L. (2012). *The Norton series on interpersonal neurobiology. The archaeology of mind: Neuroevolutionary origins of human emotion.* New York, NY, US: W. W. Norton & Company.

Perry, B., and Szalavitz, M. (2006). *The boy who was raised as a dog: And other stories from a child psychiatrist's notebook; What traumatised children can teach us about loss, love & healing.* New York: Basic Books.

Roszak, T., Gomes, M.E., and Kanner, A.D. (1995). *Ecopsychology: Restoring the earth, healing the mind.* San Francisco, CA: Sierra Club Books.

Rothschild, B. (2000). *The body remembers: The psychophysiology of trauma and trauma treatment.* New York and London: W.W. Norton & Company.

Sabini, M. (2002). *The earth has a soul: Technology & modern life.* Berkeley, CA: North Atlantic Books.

Schore, A.N. (2010). Relational trauma and the developing right brain: The neurobiology of broken attachments. In Baradon, T. (Ed.), *Relational trauma in infancy: Psychoanalytic, attachment and neuropsychological contributions to parent-infant psychotherapy* (pp. 19–47). London and New York: Routledge.

Shepard, P. (1998). *Nature and madness*. Athens, GA: University of Georgia Press.

Sholt, M., and Gavron, T. (2006). Therapeutic qualities of clay-work in art therapy and psychotherapy. A review. *Art Therapy: Journal of the American Art Therapy Association*, 23 (2), pp. 66–72.

Snir, S., and Regev, D. (2013). A dialog with five art materials: Creators share their art making experiences. *The Arts in Psychotherapy*, 40, pp. 94–100.

Stern, D. (2002). *The first relationship: Infant and mother*. Cambridge: Harvard University Press.

Trevarthen, C. (1993). The self born in intersubjectivity: The psychology of an infant communicating. In Neisser, U. (Ed.), *The perceived self: Ecological and interpersonal sources of self-knowledge* (pp. 120–173). London: Cambridge University Press.

Van der Heide, N. (2012). The art of regulation: Therapeutic action in the shared implicit relationship. *International Journal of Psychoanalytic Self Psychology*, 7 (1), pp. 29–44.

Weller, A., and Feldman, R. (2003). Emotion regulation and touch in infants: The role of cholecystokinin and opioids. *Peptides*, 24, pp. 779–788.

White, R. (2004). *Young children's relationship with nature: Its importance to children's development and the earth's future*. White Hutchinson Leisure & Learning Group.

Wilson, E.O. (1986). *Biophilia*. Cambridge, MA: Harvard University Press.

4

EARTHWAYS

Environmental arts therapy for repairing
insecure attachment and developing
creative response-ability in
an insecure world

Lia Ponton

> *Geoff stops walking and stands in front of a tall, mature ash tree grow-*
> *ing at the edge of the path in the upper woods. He stands for some*
> *moments, silently contemplating it. He verbally expresses his admiration.*
> *I gently encourage him to touch the tree first with his hands. "This is very*
> *intimate", he says "I feel this tree is definitely female. She is very strong".*
> *I invite Geoff to lean on the tree; to feel his back and spine supported*
> *by the trunk. "This feels good", he says with his eyes closed, "I feel an*
> *attachment". I then suggest experimenting with how it feels to have the*
> *front of his body in contact with the tree, with his arms wrapped around*
> *the trunk. "My son would say I was a tree hugger!" he admits, without*
> *allowing this concern to interrupt the physical experience of intimacy*
> *with the tree. Later on, Geoff tells me that he has never before allowed*
> *himself to have this kind of embodied connection with a tree and tells me*
> *that it was difficult to leave "her".*

"I know it's a cliché, but it is . . . Mother Nature. Yeah . . . I felt it."
— *(Geoff, session 3)*

In this chapter I explore some of the ways that creative engagement with our
environment facilitated by an attachment-informed environmental arts therapy
approach can support individuals to experience a sense of their interdependence
with all of life, leading to increased psychological security ('I am safe', 'I belong')

and the development of an expanded sense of self. I consider how this may enable individuals to cope better with their anxieties about the uncertain future they face – both personally in their lives and collectively as humans facing climate change and other planetary threats together – as well as how we might begin to respond to these uncertainties with courage and creativity. I will end by asking some questions about how we are responding to the threats posed to us at this time on our planet and the complex challenges that these threat responses present to us as people and as therapists.

Geoff's tree was in a wood, which is part of the natural environment where I work. This environment and everything in it is not only my partner in my work with clients but so many other things too – support, inspiration, challenge – and it is this environment which shapes my writing.

EarthWays at Holbeam

Holbeam is a pocket of land in South Devon, bordered by the River Lemon. From a small lane, a gateway leads to a five-acre meadow, which is steeply sloped until it levels out and reaches the alders, hazels and oaks lining the riverbank. A line of ash, elder, holly, hawthorn and gorse form a border into a six-acre ancient woodland, framed by conifer plantations and the river. There is a gate into the woods in the corner of the field. There is a wide track that runs alongside the river at the bottom of the woods and there are various steps and pathways up into the trees.

As we move through this environment we will also move through aspects of human attachment, developmental and psychological processes and through elements of environmental arts therapy practice. We will begin in the field, go through the gateway and into the woods. We will feel what is low down in the river and on the muddy banks, then make our way up through the woods to the higher path. Once there we will return along the path at the top of the woods until we get to a stile that leads back into the field. At the stile we will see that our view of the field has changed. We will be able to see the whole field from up here and as we step over the stile and into the field, we will begin to ask questions about how the field is impacting us as people and as therapists. Three of my clients will join us on this EarthWays exploration; they are Heather, Geoff and Eva and I am very grateful to them for allowing me to share pieces of their stories here.

The field: love, attachment and loss

We've opened the gate and come into the field; wild grasses bend in the wind. In spring and summer, pink campions, dandelions, herb Robert, speedwell and buttercups make the grass sparkle with colour. All year round, thistles and nettles may unnerve the bare-footed explorer . . .

The field we are endeavouring to explore is one in which both people and planet are experiencing distress. At its centre is the belief that as social beings with social brains (Holmes, 2014), our physiological, psychological and emotional responses to life in the world are shaped by our experiences of love, attachment and loss, and this is what all therapy (and possibly environmental activism) is primarily concerned with. This requires us to explore the field of attachment theory.

Essentially, attachment theory considers the intersubjective relationship between a child and their primary caregiver(s). A primary caregiver's capacity to provide experiences for the child which cumulatively result in a secure attachment is how the infant experiences the caregiver's love; in other words, attachments are the arteries through which love is carried. Anything which blocks or hinders the experiencing of love through this intersubjective process is experienced as loss by the child. This loss, or the threat of such a loss, produces a response in the child that has profound impact on its developing being (Baylin and Hughes, 2016). We can call this response *separation distress* (Pankseep, 2014).

Recent psychological and neuro-scientific research (Siegel, 2011a; Schore, 2009; Cozolino, 2017) has corroborated Winnicott's theory of Object Relations (1960) which proposed that the primary attachment relationship of mother and child exerts the single most decisive influence over how a person develops. The research also supports Bowlby's (1988) findings which indicated that excessive early separation experiences, poor parental bonding and insufficient co-regulation of feelings can leave individuals susceptible to particular future psychopathologies, often caused by and compounding feelings of low self-worth and a profound mistrust of intimate relationships (Wallin, 2007).

My own mother experienced post-natal depression during my first year and a half of life. She was either unable to come to me and comfort me in my distress, expressed anger towards me, or found that she did not feel the love that she had expected to feel as she held me in her arms. My memories are of a largely happy childhood, so I confess I experienced a sense of relief when she told me about my baby days, as I began to gain insight into what might lie behind the symptoms I had experienced at different times throughout my childhood, adolescence and adult life; anxiety, depression, panic attacks, irritable bowel syndrome, risk-taking behaviours and a difficulty to trust in my relationships. I understood that it was possible I had experienced a kind of attachment trauma stemming from "being left psychologically alone in unbearable emotional pain" (Allen, 2013, p. xxii).

As babies we seek both physical and psychological safety and security. We need both. We may survive if only our physical needs are met, but if our early attachment experiences were inadequate in meeting our psychological needs we are often left with psychological insecurities and unhealthy regulation tactics (Schaffer, 2004).

The dark woods and the river of feeling: body and emotion

We've stepped through the gateway and into the woods. The sunlight filters through the trees and there is constant background sound of flowing water and bird song. Here, we will begin to explore the work of environmental arts therapy in repairing insecure attachment . . .

My passion for, and belief in, the work of environmental arts therapy arises from the diminishment of my own attachment trauma symptoms experienced through working creatively with the other-than-human world, either 'alone' or with other people.

What was Geoff feeling when he embraced the ash tree? And what is it that I feel every time I allow my body to make contact with the rough bark of an old oak tree or a slender weeping willow? How can these embodied experiences support reparation of insecure attachment symptoms?

Down by the river – the body

We are down by the riverbank now, in the soft mud, amongst the roots of the trees. The smell is of damp earth; down here fungi swells in shades of brown, orange and white. Here we explore what happens in our bodies when we are babies and when we are grown, and how working with our bodies can help us reduce feelings of insecurity . . .

Scientific studies have shown that spending time outdoors generates feelings of well-being and a reduction in stress (Tsunetsugu et al., 2010; Bratman et al., 2014). For me this is experienced as a deep exhalation; it feels as if all my body systems are slowing down to enable a sense of peace. I pay attention to what happens in my body when I walk through ancient woodland, sit next to a stream or lie down on a hillside and look up at the clouds as they travel across the sky. I notice a sense of well-being.

Every 'body' I have welcomed through the gateway at EarthWays has described the sense of calm and wellness that being in this environment generates in them:

This feels safe. This feels nurturing.

(Heather, session 1)

A feeling of safety is generally considered to be a therapeutic necessity and creating this feeling within the therapeutic encounter can be a long and complex process. Within environmental arts therapy there is a richness to this process, and the intensity of finding safety in the one-to-one human relationship is lessened due to additional holding from the environment.

> Eva sits in her 'womb space'; a place in the field, next to the gorse bushes that she often returns to. She tells me that she feels safe there; she feels held and calm. She can reflect on what has been, simply 'be' and give her body the time it needs to readjust to feeling safe and well.

Once people feel this sense of safety they become able to allow authentic emotional responses to stimuli to come through their bodies. We perceive reality through the body and its senses. The emotions that we feel in our bodies in response to what we perceive through our senses shape our reality. As young infants our emotions are the only way that we understand our reality, (Siegel, 2011a) and our bodies are the primary means of communication between self and other. Where there is lack of attachment communication the body is directly and adversely impacted and our capacity to regulate emotions is compromised; emotions are experienced only as physical sensations, and those physical sensations become our reality (Wallin, 2007; Van der Kolk, 2015).

Environmental arts therapy can support clients to experience lasting change by activating the sensory, bodily experience of emotions (Levine, 2010). Working in nature means working with the physical world and, therefore, by default the body and the senses in relation to the physical world. Nature *is* physical and in environmental arts therapy it is interacted with, providing us with a physical, embodied, sensory experience of our inner and outer world. Because environmental arts therapy is active, using techniques from both drama and art therapy, it involves "the way the self is realised by and through the body," and this results in a "deepened encountering of the material the client brings to therapy" (Jones, 2007, p. 113).

> Geoff is walking up through the trees following a short pause where I guided him through a body scan, to help connect him with all of himself. As he walks, he seems gently surprised and says, "I can feel my strength and power", "feel the health of my body" and "feel connected to my body and the strength of my muscles" as they support him to climb the steep bank.

In the river – the flow of feeling

> The cool water of the river surges and glides gently around the rocks and stones on the riverbed, non-stop on its journey from the moor. We

> *lower ourselves into the water and feel our body's response to the flow*
> *of the stream . . .*

I was struck when two of the clients in this chapter described having a river at the bottom of their gardens, and the third lived by the sea. They all talked about these bodies of water as being a significant part of their lives and described them in terms of both attachment and healing. In many cultures and traditions water is associated with healing and with feelings. My clients will often sit by the water, create pieces of art with the stones on the river bed, or hold rituals where the water helps to carry things away or show them which way to go.

Environmental arts therapy values expression of experience through action and emotion, as well as thought and voice. Working with emotion is fundamental within an attachment-orientated approach, since attachment relationships are the context within which our emotions are both validated and regulated (Fonagy et al., 2005; Schore, 2003).

> During a ritual to let go of feelings long held, and physically working with earth, fire, feather and stone, Eva suddenly realises that her long-held sadness and anger come from an experience of loss; a previous therapist who had 'left her'. Tears form and fall softly as she says words that she had not known needed to be spoken.

The ascent through the woods: encounter, play, myth and ritual

> *We are walking up the steps that lead through the woods. Depending on*
> *the time of year the forest floor may be carpeted with pungent-smelling*
> *wild garlic and bluebells, or the crisp red, brown, gold of fallen leaves.*
> *The trees surround us, tower above us, seeking out the light. Our emo-*
> *tions are witnessed and given form and dialogue by both the human and*
> *non-human that we encounter, engaging the different parts of our brain*
> *that are associated with attachment and offering opportunity for repair . . .*

The encounter with the other

We learn to regulate our emotions through the experience of intersubjectivity. This involves a discovery of one another and the development of the self in relationship with the other. The three aspects of intersubjectivity are shared affect (or emotional attunement), shared intention and shared attention. Environmental arts therapy offers many opportunities for intersubjectivity based in nonverbal experience. Attunement within the client-therapist and client-environment relationships is likely to activate mirror neurons and the other parts of the brain that were most active in the initial attachment relationship (the amygdala, hippocampus and structures underlying the cortex).

> Heather and I lie side by side on the hillside; the land rising up to hold us both as we let go into it; she more than me I hope, as it is my role to hold her there too. The sun shines on our faces. She lets out a deep sigh, which I mirror more subtly to let her know I am there, feeling it with her.

Many people, including indigenous teachers, ecopsychologists and ecotherapists, view the Earth as a living entity; not an object, but "subject, animated matter, materializing spirit" (Mies, 2014, p. 161) or a subject with soul (Berry, 1990; Vaughan-Lee, 2005; Jung in Sabini, 2002). Often our relationship with the Earth is viewed metaphorically as a mother/child relationship. This is a complex metaphor, which some view as being unhelpful.

Seager says "if the Earth is our mother, then we are children and cannot be held fully accountable for our actions" (Seager, 1994, p. 201). But children are also full of love, care and wonder and so could potentially make healthy, loving and responsible choices in service of the Earth – as proven by the courageous actions of 16-year-old climate activist Greta Thunberg. Also, as we grow it often becomes the child's responsibility to care for the parent when they are too sick or frail to care for themselves. This accountability broadens the metaphor moving beyond dependence into reciprocity.

Roszak suggests that our "relations extend beyond family and society to embrace the natural world that sustains us all" (Roszak, 2001, p. 293). Consequently, when clients are supported to experience feelings of maternal care from the natural world as primary caregiver, separation distress may be soothed and transformed. Baker (2013) suggests that in this way recognising our dependence on the natural world can become a source of strength.

When Geoff embraces the tree, Heather lays on the earth and Eva sits in her 'womb space', there is a sense that the world accepts and loves them, and that they accept and love the world in return.

Studies into attachment and child development have shown that infants respond to very subtle changes in their surroundings and can detect when their caregiver is anxious, detached or upset. Peter Wohlleben, in his book *The Hidden Life of Trees* (2016), suggests that we humans are equipped with intuitive ways of acknowledging and responding to the state of our surroundings, i.e. whether we are in a safe place and whether the surroundings themselves are healthy. He tells us that not only have scientific studies shown that people feel calmer among trees in general but also that blood pressure rises when one is among conifers which have been planted in environments that are too warm and dry (resulting in trees that are thirsty and unstable), whereas blood pressure falls amongst healthy oaks in their native habitat. We respond to the health of our environment, and for our nervous system to be calm we need all of our caregivers (human and not human) to be able to thrive. This raises many questions about what happens to us when we live in a damaged environment, especially with the knowledge that we may be partly responsible for that damage.

However, if we do therapy work in a healthy natural environment, we are supported by a real biochemical ally in the therapeutic process, one that helps to soothe the nervous system of our clients. Working in nature also provides additional witnessing; witnessing that is unbound by the limits of human tolerance for emotional release. Mother Nature can offer a profound experience of unconditional acceptance of emotion, providing synchronistic natural mirroring of the client's emotional experience just as it is needed. The therapist works with the client in noticing this – such as pointing out the ducklings that appear around the corner just as Geoff expresses his longing for something new, or noticing with Eva that she sits in a cramped uncomfortable position upon rocky, sloping ground as she describes "the uncomfortable place" of feelings such as despair, jealousy and resentment.

These experiences, once trusted, tend to become self-perpetuating and may help repair any lack of provision of attunement and witnessing in a person's initial human attachment relationship.

Play

Jennings (2011) argues that attachment is, by its very nature, playful. She describes how the complex neurochemical processes that constitute parental bonding and the child's development of a sense of self and place in the world are established through different kinds of play.

Geoff found the most freedom from 'being in his head' – which he described as a dam blocking the flow of feeling – when we established that everything that happened when he passed through the gateway into the wood could be an experiment. "If it is an experiment, then you cannot fail", I reminded him. Developmental transformations, a form of dramatherapy pioneered by David Read Johnson (1991), also establishes that everything that happens within the therapy time and space is a play space; there is mutual agreement that everything that goes on is a representation of real or imagined being. This allows for experimentation and the freedom that comes from the ambivalent experience of both 'being' and 'not being' and is a quality I welcome in my work.

> Geoff said he did not feel comfortable with the word play, but he was happy with the word experiment. In this experimental session, he took hold of great

long strands of ivy and swung them back and forth as far as he could. I joined him. Later, he began to launch great, long dead sticks through the air like spears watching and hearing them crash and splinter against other trees or the woodland floor. All this happened without words, but with open smiles and twinkling eyes, and later, quiet and fierce determination.

This permission to experiment seemed to enable Geoff to experience himself in a way that he had not before, opening up new possibilities and releasing his capacity for transformation (Emunah and Johnson, 2009).

Stuart Brown defines play as "an absorbing, apparently purposeless activity that provides enjoyment and a suspension of self-consciousness and sense of time" (Brown, 2009, p. 60). Maslow (1962) suggested that the full absorption and openness required in play is one of the ways that individuals can move towards self-actualisation. Among other freedoms, play provides us with the opportunity to recognise and grow the healthy parts of ourselves so that we can strengthen our capacity to comfort and repair the damaged parts.

"I'd like to make something", Heather says. We walk up the steps at the side of the wood and she sits. She gathers wilted, fragile looking ransoms – long gone the days when they provided a pungent scent and robust green leaves – and threads the delicate strands onto a twig. She is absorbed for over twenty minutes. When she turns to me to invite me back in, I comment that the creation looks like a child's mobile. There follows an exploration of motherhood and from this the grief of miscarriage naturally flows.

In my experience, this kind of playful absorption is like a form of meditation. The activity is not designed to distract, rather it provides an opportunity for the unconscious to be brought into the light and given form. Because the activity is playful, spontaneous and creative, there is a lightness and space around it. This is where we can compare the engagement with personal process that we might experience during meditation (Gammage, 2017).

I have a distinct memory from my childhood. I was five or six years old and playing an imaginary game with two of my classmates in a wild corner of the vast school playing fields. Something else caught their interest, but I couldn't be torn away from the game; I was too committed to it to leave. Quickly, two large trees supplanted my friends and I assigned these trees roles in the game as my parents. I hugged each tree and said "goodbye mum", "goodbye dad" before going off on an imaginary adventure alone. The two trees were my safe place, my secure base, and I returned to them again and again with tales of how my adventures were progressing. The trees were solid and unmoving; generous and somehow affectionate. They made me feel good. They made me feel loved.

As Wohlleben (2016) has explored, it is likely that very real physical and biochemical interactions were taking place when I played with the two tree parents. At the same time, I was behaving *as if* the tree was my caregiver. As Jennings (2011) explains, the brain does not know the difference between a real lived experience and an imagined 'as if' experience. This is why dramatic enactment or any experiences which allow for an expansion of our reality using the 'as if' of the imagination can have a real impact on our brain functioning and hence on reparation of unsatisfactory attachment experiences.

Ritual and myth

Eva selects a flowering female of the lords-and-ladies plant to represent her mother. It is August and the berries have mostly dropped. She describes the plant as being exuberant and a little grotesque; something which draws your attention but is actually decaying. Eva then places other members of her family around this matriarchal stem and is able to relate difficult stories from her past and present about her relationship with her mother and other members of the family.

The emotional distance achieved by creating this constellation and projecting her family members onto 'objects' and organisms in the wood enabled Eva to tell her stories. It also allowed her to have a physical relationship with those stories that enabled her to stay present with them and to express her feelings around them. When talking about her difficult, almost overwhelming feelings, she looked up and around the wood and said "I can put them here. There's somewhere for them to go". In our sessions, Eva referred back to the normal 'white walls' of therapy rooms and how the physical space had not enabled her to relax; she would often dissociate rather than engage in her process. Since the brain instinctively prioritises security over exploration, it is likely that this was a way of protecting herself from hyperactivation of the nervous system. The kind of projective work that Eva did in the woods allowed her to express her feelings in a way that was contained and did not result in emotional flooding and therefore disassociation; she found herself able to 'stay in the uncomfortable place'.

This way of working contained elements of ritual, and ritual was something that Eva came back to week after week. In an early session she released sycamore seeds into the stream as a way of saying goodbye to people she had cared for who had died. Her most significant loss was of a friend who had died when she was just a teenager. The seed representing this friend refused to go downstream and swirled around and around in an eddy making Eva smile. She drew meaning from the experience, enjoying having her friend be playful, refusing to do what was asked and instead staying close to her – reflecting how the memory of her friend and the loss of her had been with her throughout her life.

Rituals allow for the processing of difficult feelings in a way that is safely contained. We know that during a ritual there will be a beginning, middle and an end, and this enables us to allow feelings to arise, be released and then moved on from, however terrifying they may be in normal circumstances. Rituals have been used for individual and community healing and transformation in indigenous communities for millennia, and their use in our therapy work now can lead to clients feeling a sense of control and influence over their lives (Berger and Mcleod, 2006). Campbell (2005) describes ritual as an enactment of a myth – the mythology of the psyche. When the individual participates in a ritual they are brought into connection with their personal mythology and the wisdom contained within it.

Kerényi describes mythology as a phenomenon which "in profundity, permanence, and universality is comparable only with nature herself" (Kerényi, 1985, p. 1). Embodied experience of ritual and myth enables people to make meaning and experience transformation, develop resilience and feel more courageous. Myths contain the entire gamut of human emotions and archetypes and hence are rich material for working with insecure clients. Metaphors contained within myth enable clients to see who they are/have been/and could become, and this can strengthen their capacity to create narratives for their own lives. Combining this with the natural object reality of the therapy space (for example, a tree trunk to act as Bran's bridge over to Ireland to rescue his sister Branwyn from the cruel king) means that myths and metaphors are given physical form and can be interacted with physically. This provides sensory as well as neurological memories just like the memories formed in infancy.

The path out of the woods: mindfulness, mentalisation, meta-awareness and reflection

We are walking along the top path in the woods now, back towards the field. We can see the crowns of some of the trees below us and the flowing river at the bottom of the valley. We look back and see where we have come from. We notice the impact our experiences have had on us and reflect on their meaning in our lives . . .

Supporting clients to develop an awareness of their words, actions, thoughts and feelings, as well as the happenings in the object world that they are in relationship with, supports the process of mentalisation and development of a reflective stance. To some extent, all therapists are concerned with the slowing down of psychological processes in order to help people notice, question, and challenge or accept their habitual thoughts, feelings and patterns of behaviour. Working in nature supports a mindful stance, a slowing down of the process of being, since the sensory experience of being outdoors means it is less easy to become preoccupied or dissociated, as Eva testified when she remembered with a shudder the white walls of previous therapeutic interventions.

Symbols and metaphors found within nature evoke thoughts, feelings and memories linking the conscious and the unconscious. This supports clients to develop meta-awareness of their experience and to link thought with feeling. This is essential to integration and to healing the pathological self-regulation tactics that result from caregivers having been unable to provide co-regulation when the child is distressed (Holmes, 2014). These tactics, inherent to insecure attachment patterns of behaviour, often cause minimization or denial of experience (in the dismissing state of mind) or overwhelm (in the preoccupied state of mind) (Main, 1991). Wallin argues that "the more we are able to mobilize a reflective stance, the more resilient we will be" (Wallin, 2007, p. 4). He adds: "*To the extent that we make it possible for patients to mentalize, we strengthen their ability to regulate their affects, to integrate experiences that have been dissociated, and to feel a more solid, coherent sense of self*" (Wallin, 2007, p. 4).

To be able to experience mentalisation and meta-awareness, clients need to learn how to pay non-judgemental attention to their emotional experience at any given time. They need to develop a mindful stance towards their inner and outer experience (as does the therapist).

Geoff stands on the top path and looks out through a circle of trees to the open countryside. "I feel wonderful" he says. I ask: "What does wonderful feel like?" Geoff closes his eyes and describes what is happening in his body and mind.

Paying attention to sensory stimulation outside the body can also support us to pay gentle attention to the sensory, bodily feelings that are happening inside us – something Van der Kolk (2015) terms "interrospection". This has benefits related to bodily and affective regulation, attuned communication, insight and empathy, which research has shown to be associated with secure attachment (Siegel, 2011b). In environmental arts therapy internal feelings are often projected out onto nature and given form or voice and so the client's capacity to mentalise and take a reflective stance towards their experience – which is essential to creating therapeutic change (Wallin, 2007) – is further strengthened.

The complex reality of nature is often reflective of our own complex inner nature, and in environmental arts therapy we notice these reflections as a form of validation and to support the client's change process. Scull argues that the natural world is "not a metaphor for the human condition" instead "it is very real and very complex" (Scull, 2009, p. 147) and should be responded to in kind. This is certainly true, but by allowing our projections and using aspects of nature as symbols and metaphors for our human experiences we are encouraged towards a greater sense of wonder and gratitude for all that nature provides and hence towards a more caring and responsible attitude. Once people can see themselves within the natural world they experience an embodied sense of being a part of nature and not separate from it. I believe, like many of my teachers, that developing a culture of witness and appreciation within the therapeutic encounter with nature is fundamental to cultivate lasting inner and outer change, in conversation with Banks and Prentice (2015) and Macy and Brown (2014). Expanding empathic identification may result in increased empathy for self (self-compassion) and hence support the healing of core emotional wounds and increased identification with nature. This tenderness towards self and the world is essential to creating a new way of being in and with the world.

Seeing the field 'through new eyes': empathic identification and expansion of the self

We're at the stile now, high up in the woods looking out at the field. The field looks different; the seasons have changed. Things have grown and been let go of . . .

Intersubjective experiences with the natural world can help to expand the sense of self; to experience oneself as an 'ecological self' (Macy, 2009). When this happens, we experience ourselves as a part of all that lives, therefore worthy of love, safe and held by Mother Nature, who – as a congruent caregiver – reflects the self back to us. The self is developed in a specifically relational context, which includes the object world so that clients can experience transformation through relationship. This approach to therapy agrees with object relations psychology but goes further and includes the other-than-human.

Griffiths (2014) suggests that children are embedded in a present experience that includes their original self, their expanding social world, their affinity to nature and their relationship with the space they live within. They are what Conn and Conn term "open to the other" (Conn and Conn, 2009, p. 112), which includes all of life. There are many who suggest that in the West, our sense of being embedded in the world has all but disappeared. In pre-modern and indigenous cultures the enchantment of childhood was not seen as a naïve phase prior to adulthood. Growth is supported through initiation rites and rituals that include, rather than reject, participation with the natural world. Roszak (2001) suggests that for meaningful change to happen in the inner and outer worlds, a form of therapy is required that supports people to experience a child's 'enchanted sense of the world' once again.

Eva asks me: "Have you seen the beautiful blue rock in the stream by the bridge?" She tells me with enthusiasm about a sparkling blue rock that sits in the fast-flowing water. Her eyes glisten and she seems full of a sense of wonder as she describes the rock in great detail. I share in her sense of awe and reverence; I too want to see the rock and delight in her delight.

Eva is developing a receptive, spontaneous way of being and a deep relationship with nature, embedded in the present, is emerging in her. Winter says that as we begin to experience this embeddedness in "an emotionally meaningful way, our sense of self changes" (Winter, 1996, p. 249). This expansion of the sense of self allows people to cultivate greater flexibility, a wider range of responses to lived experiences and an improved capacity to cope with instability.

If we can expand our sense of self to include the cosmos (a transpersonal view) and develop the embedded understanding that our identity is in relationship with the larger ecosystem of which we are a part, we can naturally develop the identification needed to act in service of all of life (which is no longer experienced as separate from us).

The benefits of this identification are reciprocal, as Jordan and Hinds explain in their introduction to *Ecotherapy Theory, Research and Practice* (2016). If we can feel empathy for the orangutans being made homeless in the Indonesian rainforests due to palm oil extraction, perhaps we can then feel tenderness for ourselves whatever our predicament may be which in turn may lead to a strengthening of courage to act on behalf of the orangutans. This empathic identification can continue on a feedback loop providing us with the love and courage we need to keep going in our own lives and to find the creative responses we need to act on behalf of all of life.

The gift of being human is our capacity to create, to relate, to reason and to play. Environmental arts therapy honours each individual expression of this humanness which is viewed as an aspect of nature expressing itself.

After spending a significant portion of her session talking through some difficult experiences, I invite Eva to spend her remaining time making something without thinking about it. She goes to a corner of the wood and works with all her focus and energy. After just a few minutes, she presents an exquisite 'magical imp', with acorn head and sycamore crown. The imp has several magical powers but essentially is playful, spontaneous, loving, creative and 'impish'.

The magic imp (Figure 4.1) provides Eva with other ways of responding to the people and situations in her life; it shows her the creative possibilities that are available to her.

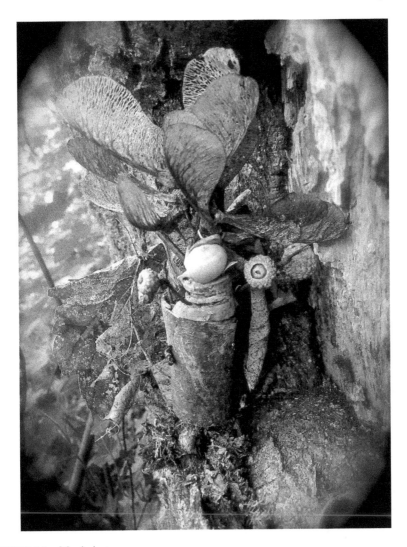

FIGURE 4.1   Magic imp

Returning to the field with another perspective

We are back in the field. We have changed and so has the field. Here we see the current state of the world and wonder how we will respond creatively to it . . .

As humans we have a fundamental preoccupation with survival (physical) and security (psychological). Advances in science and technology have enabled many of us to become aware of local and global problems that threaten both of these fundamental concerns – many of which, such as climate change, seem to exceed our coping capacities (Weintrobe, 2013; Adams, 2014).

We are bearing witness to on-going destruction of habitats including vital rainforests, exploitation of fossil fuels and mass extinction of species (See World Wildlife Foundation [WWF], 2018). Since publication of the latest Intergovernmental Panel on Climate Change (IPCC) (2018) report in October 2018, the media has begun to describe climate change as a global emergency and activists are pressing for local and central governments to do the same. British national newspaper *The Guardian* (2018) holds the editorial position that climate change poses "an existential threat to the human race" a line which has been taken by many for many years (Klein, 2014). According to Joanna Macy (2014) the "loss of certainty for the on-goingness of life is the pivotal psychological reality of our time". Psychologically, this results in anxiety, cognitive dissonance, denial and disavowal, amongst other complex and uncomfortable feelings. I personally have been rocked with despair and anxiety over the situation that humanity faces, making it difficult to carry on with the tasks of daily life. And yet at some point the headlines disappear from view and life somehow moves forward with 'business as usual'.

Are we exhibiting dismissive, avoidant and ambivalent attachment behaviours towards our primary caregiver, the Earth? Like the insecure child, we seem to be stuck in the paradox of denying our dependence, whilst also experiencing an abiding preoccupation that what we depend upon will be withdrawn from us (Bowlby, 1988). Do we disengage because of the difficult feelings this insecure attachment evokes? Are we witnessing collective withdrawal and disengagement from ourselves and others, including nature, because of anxiety-inducing feelings?

As therapists we face unprecedented challenges brought about by this psychological reality. We need to ask ourselves how we can work creatively with these challenges. For me this has involved developing a model of resourcing that supports me to keep engaging and to trust my creative responses. This begins with developing wonder, intimacy, trust, playfulness, mindfulness and reflective practices in my relationship with all of life – human and not human – as described in this chapter. It involves developing the capacity to love, and the resilience to cope with loss by honouring it through feeling it. It involves holding the view of the field in mind as I work with people of all ages to help them restore their trust in themselves and in others. There is little that is more important at this time in the world than participating in supporting people to engage with what really matters and to do so in a way that is beautiful and true.

References

Adams, M. (2014). Inaction and environmental crisis: Narrative, defence mechanisms and the social organisation of denial. *Psychoanalysis, Culture & Society*, 19 (1), pp. 52–71.

Allen, J.G. (2013). *Restoring mentalizing in attachment relationships: Treating trauma with plain old therapy*. Washington, DC: American Psychiatric Publishing.

Baker, C. (2013). *Collapsing consciously*. Berkeley, CA: North Atlantic Books.

Banks, S., and Prentice, H. (2015). Conversation with Lia Ponton, 26 April.

Baylin, J., and Hughes, D. (2016). *The neurobiology of attachment-focused therapy: Enhancing connection & trust in the treatment of children & adolescents*. New York: W.W. Norton & Company.

Berger, R., and McLeod, J. (2006). Incorporating nature into therapy: A framework for practice. *Journal of Systemic Therapies*, 25 (2), pp. 80–94.

Berry, T. (1990). *Dream of the earth* (Reprint edition). Berkeley, CA: University of California Press.

Bowlby, J. (1988). *A secure base*. Abingdon: Routledge.

Bratman, G.N., Hamilton, J.P., Hahn, K.S., Daily, G.C., and Gross, J.J. (2014). Nature experience reduces rumination and subgenual prefrontal cortex activation. *PNAS*, 112 (28), pp. 8567–8572.

Brown, S. (2009). *Play: How it shapes the brain, opens the imagination, and invigorates the soul*. New York: Avery Penguin Group.

Campbell, J. (2005). *The wisdom of Joseph Campbell*. New Dimensions radio interview with Michael Toms, Hay House (Audio CD).

Conn, L., and Conn, S. (2009). Opening to the other. In Buzzel, C., and Chalquist, C. (Eds.), *Ecotherapy: Healing with nature in mind* (pp. 111–115). San Francisco, CA: Sierra Club Books.

Cozolino, L. (2017). *The neuroscience of psychotherapy: Healing the social brain* (Norton series on interpersonal neurobiology). New York: W.W. Norton & Company.

Emunah, R., and Read Johnson, D. (2009). The current state of the field of dramatherapy. In Read-Johnson, D., and Emunah, R. (Eds.), *Current approaches in dramatherapy* (2nd edition, pp. 24–33). Springfield, IL: Charles C Thomas Pub Ltd.

Fonagy, P., Gyorgy, G., Jurist, E., and Target, M. (Eds.). (2005). *Affect regulation, mentalization, and the development of the self* (New edition). New York: Karnac Books.

Gammage, D. (2017). *Playful awakening: Releasing the gift of play in your life*. London: Jessica Kingsley Publishers.

Griffiths, J. (2014). *Kith: The riddle of the childscape*. London: Penguin.

Holmes, J. (2014). *The neuroscience of attachment*. Video. Retrieved from: https://vimeo.com/88343229.

Intergovernmental Panel on Climate Change (IPCC). (2018). *Summary for policymakers of IPCC special report on global warming of 1.5°C approved by governments*. Retrieved from: www.ipcc.ch/sr15/chapter/summary-for-policy-makers/.

Jennings, S. (2011). *Healthy attachments and neuro-dramatic-play*. London: Jessica Kingsley Publishers.

Jones, P. (2007). *Drama as therapy. Theory, practice and research* (2nd edition). Hove: Routledge.

Jordan, M., and Hinds, J. (2016). *Ecotherapy theory, research and practice*. London: Palgrave.

Kerényi, C. (1985). Prolegomena. In Jung, C.G., and Kerényi, C. (Eds.), *The science of mythology. Essays on the myth of the divine child and the mysteries of Eleusis* (Revised edition, pp. 1–28). Abingdon: Routledge.

Klein, N. (2014). *This changes everything. Capitalism vs. the climate*. New York: Simon and Schuster.

Levine, P.A. (2010). *In an unspoken voice: How the body releases trauma and restores goodness*. Berkeley, CA: North Atlantic Books.

Macy, J. (2009). The greening of the self. In Buzzel, C., and Chalquist, C. (Eds.), *Ecotherapy: Healing with nature in mind* (pp. 238–245). San Francisco, CA: Sierra Club Books.

Macy, J. (2014). *Joanna Macy and the great turning*. Directed by Chris Landry. Retrieved from: www.joannamacyfilm.org/.

Macy, J., and Brown, M. (2014). *Coming back to life: The updated guide to the work that reconnects*. Gabriola Island, Canada: New Society Publishers.

Main, M. (1991). Metacognitive knowledge, metacognitive monitoring, and singular (coherent) vs. multiple (incoherent) models of attachment: Some findings and some directions for future research. In Marris, P., Stevenson-Hinde, J., and Parkes, C. (Eds.), *Attachment across the life cycle* (pp. 127–159). New York: Routledge.

Maslow, A.H. (1962). *Toward a psychology of being*. Princeton: D. Van Nostrand Company.

Mies, M. (2014). White man's dilemma: His search for what he has destroyed. In Mies, M., and Shiva, V. (Eds.), *Ecofeminism* (2nd edition, pp. 132–163). London: Zed Books.

Pankseep, J. (2014). *The science of emotions*. Talk at TEDxRainier. Retrieved from: http://tedx talks.ted.com/video/The-science-of-emotions-Jaak-Pa;search%3AThe%20science%20 of%20emotions.

Read-Johnson, D. (1991). The theory and technique of transformations in drama therapy. *The Arts in Psychotherapy*, 18 (4), pp. 285–300.

Roszak, T. (2001). *The voice of the earth* (2nd edition). Grand Rapids, MI: Phanes Press Inc.

Sabini, M. (Ed.). (2002). *The earth has a soul: C.G. Jung's writings on nature, technology and modern life*. Berkeley, CA: North Atlantic Books.

Schaffer, H.R. (2004). *Introducing child psychology*. London: Blackwell.

Schore, A. (2003). *Affect regulation and the repair of the self*. New York: W.W. Norton & Company.

Schore, A. (2009). The paradigm shift: The right brain and the relational unconscious. In *Plenary address: American psychological association, 2009 annual convention*. PowerPoint. Retrieved from: www.allanschore.com/pdf/SchoreAPAPlenaryFinal09.pdf.

Scull, J. (2009). Tailoring nature therapy to the client. In Buzzel, C., and Chalquist, C. (Eds.), *Ecotherapy: Healing with nature in mind* (pp. 140–148). San Francisco, CA: Sierra Club Books.

Seager, J. (1994). *Earth follies: Coming to feminist terms with the global environmental crisis*. New York: Routledge.

Siegel, D. (2011a). *The neurological basis of behaviour, the mind, the brain and human relationships*. Video. Retrieved from: https://youtu.be/B7kBgaZLHaA.

Siegel, D. (2011b). *On ambivalent attachment*. Video. Retrieved from: www.psychalive.org/ category/videos.

The Guardian. (2018). *The Guardian view on climate change: A global emergency*. Retrieved from: www.theguardian.com/commentisfree/2018/oct/08/the-guardian-view-on-climate-change-a-global-emergency.

Tsunetsugu, Y., Park, B-J., and Miyazaki, Y. (2010). Trends in research related to "Shinrin-yoku" (taking in the forest atmosphere or forest bathing) in Japan. *Environmental Health and Preventive Medicine*, 15 (1), pp. 27–37.

Van der Kolk, B. (2015). *The body keeps the score: Mind, brain and body in the transformation of trauma*. London: Penguin.

Vaughan-Lee, L. (2005). Anima mundi: Awakening the soul of the world. *Sufi Journal*, 67 (Autumn). Retrieved from: www.goldensufi.org/a_animamundi.html.

Wallin, D. (2007). *Attachment in psychotherapy*. New York: The Guildford Press.

Weintrobe, S. (2013). *Engaging with climate change: Psychoanalytic and interdisciplinary perspectives*. Hove: Routledge.

Winnicott, D.W. (1960). The theory of the parent-infant relationship. *International Journal of Psycho-Analysis*, 41, pp. 585–595.

Winter, D. (1996). *Ecological psychology: Healing the split between planet and self*. New York: HarperCollins.

Wohlleben, P. (2016). *The hidden life of trees*. London: William Collins.

World Wildlife Foundation (WWF). (2018). *Living planet report – 2018: Aiming higher*. In Grooten, M., and Almond, R.E.A. (Eds.). Gland, Switzerland: WWF. Retrieved from: https://wwf.panda.org/knowledge_hub/all_publications/living_planet_report_2018/.

5

BRINGING THE OUTSIDE IN

Reflecting upon Mother within a pilot group in environmental arts therapy

Michelle Edinburgh

Introduction

The idea for an environmental arts therapy group emerged during the completion of my training in this field and at a time when I was transitioning to a new art psychotherapy role and to a new city, Plymouth. I was keen to put what I had learnt into practice and my new employers agreed to support the delivery of the environmental arts therapy model. My colleague Gary Cohen, a specialist counsellor with a long-standing interest in both outdoor and creative therapies, expressed a keen desire to co-facilitate the new group with me. Thus, an eighteen-week environmental arts therapy pilot group called 'Bringing the Outside In' began to take shape.

The client group was formed of adult mental health service users with severe and enduring difficulties who had been referred to Psychotherapy Services for more in depth and longer-term support. Initially a small group of clients received a screening assessment to see if they were suitable for the group. They were all invited to join the group and after two pre-group tester sessions they all agreed to fully opt in for the full duration of the therapy.

The group was based in a medium sized therapy room within the walled grounds of Mount Gould Hospital, set within a residential area and nestled high up on a hill overlooking the River Plym estuary. Beyond this the extensive woods of the National Trust property Saltram House mark the horizon, and from the therapy room windows the changing faces of weather can be observed sweeping over the hills and houses and across the full length of the estuary. The therapy room is simply furnished with four long tables each laid along a wall, a storage cupboard for art materials and a circle of chairs set around a small, round coffee table. The entrance to the room is from the reception/waiting area, where there are also facilities for refreshments. The room is stocked with an assortment of different sizes and colours of papers, clay, water-based paints, acrylic paints, pencils, oil pastels, chalk pastels, string and glue and a collection of natural materials such as stones, pebbles, shells, sea glass and pine cones. A selection of these were laid out on the tables at the beginning of the group.

The outside of the therapy room is surrounded by a plentiful array of cultivated and non-cultivated trees and grassy borders. Most of these areas are regularly gardened, but a few remain relatively wild and overgrown with tall pines, turkey oaks, sessile oaks, red oaks, sycamores, chestnuts, rowan and many different types of saplings. Depending on the time of year cleavers, bluebells, nettles, celandine and other such plants grow abundantly in between the trees and shrubs. This outdoor space is adjacent to a small hospital car park and pedestrian walkways, but despite that the area remains quiet and is not particularly overlooked.

Each week in the morning the group members gathered together at the therapy space and spent a short time listening to the facilitators share some common seasonal themes for that particular session. Clients would often join in and share their observations upon the natural world around them. Immediately after this the group would go outside to explore and collect natural materials for approximately fifteen to twenty minutes. Materials such as leaves, flowers, blossom, feathers, berries, fruits, moss, stones and sticks were gathered and taken back to the therapy room where they were laid upon one of the tables. Members of the group were then asked to select an item for an emotional check-in. They were invited to choose something that they identified with, that reflected or symbolised some aspect of their current feelings or state of mind. Then in turn each client expressed for a few moments what it was that had drawn them to this item and shared a little of their present feelings and experience.

After this the members of the group would spend almost an hour creating an image from the available materials, both those provided in the therapy room and those gathered from outdoors. They were encouraged to follow either a personal theme that was emerging for them in the present moment or to use the guided season-related themes such as the harvest, new beginnings, light and dark or nesting. Upon completion the group returned to the circle to share feedback about what they had made, what they had discovered about themselves and how they felt. A strong emphasis was given to the expression of feelings. We have consistently found that it is in the allowing of these long-held feelings, and in having them witnessed, that a client's personal blocks begin to move and flow again, and they begin to find some relief for their unhealed wounds. Finally, the group all joined in with the tidying up and clearing away of materials. If they wished they could fill in a feedback form which allowed them to reflect critically on the session, sharing with us what they had found helpful or unhelpful and what, if anything, they might like to do differently in the future or what they might like to give more emphasis to.

Abusive mother, the inner tyrant and being unable to change

It became increasingly obvious that much anger in the group was emerging in connection to relationship or lack of relationship with mothers. Stories of failed mothering, or neglectful and abusive mothers, gradually appeared as a dominant theme. Demonic and condemning eyes, often red or green, appeared and reappeared in the images made during the course of the group. It transpired that the gaze of mother was not known to be the gentle, loving, protective and unconditional gaze that supports the foundation of a self-confident, happy and outgoing child. Time and time again we heard stories of abandonment, neglect, cruelty and criticism. Images of hateful mothers included sharp, pointed, squawking bird like masks that caricatured not only the experience of hostile mothering but also the experience of having internalised this tyrannical aspect within the self. Self-hatred and guilt often accompanied the painful realisation that mother's voice now appeared to live successfully within the self, like a ghostly harpy that would not cease its critical tirade. Clients shared strong fears of getting it wrong and hence of there being no point in really trying. It was felt that this internalised critical mother invalidates the self and 'rubbishes' whatever is created. Consequently, everything is too much or too little, never just good enough. In comparing oneself unfavourably to others, one is never allowed to fully settle into a loving acceptance of what one has, who one is, or who one might become. Clients also shared their feelings about having to be the good boy or good girl and the need to please mother in various ways. For some, attempting to be 'good' artists and complimenting others on how 'good' their images were felt both compulsory and symbolic of this. Where mother is always the other, there was a constant attempt at being liked or feeling loved, arriving out of a habit to pacify and please and to secure one's position as 'the apple of her eye'. For one client a still life depiction of a holly branch illustrated this theme. Expressing bitterness and anger, he described how he had shown artistic promise as a child but was denied the opportunity by his parents to attend art school. The prickly evergreen is drawn by him in such a way as to highlight his artistic prowess attempting perhaps to prove his worth. It appears to vigorously and aggressively fill the left-hand side of the page leaving the remaining right side empty and spacious emphasising perhaps all that was absent and unrealised.

In *Women Who Run with The Wolves,* author Clarissa Pinkola Estes recounts the story of the ugly duckling and elaborates on 'kinds of mothers' and '*the mother complex*': namely the ambivalent mother, the collapsed mother, and the child mother or the un-mothered mother. She depicts an internal mother in the psyche that duplicates the personal, childhood mother. This internal mother includes other mothering figures of our early years as well as the cultural good/bad mother images that we were exposed to at that time. She explores further '*todas las madres*', the idea of having 'many mothers' during one's lifetime as vital relationships that support the creative life. Additionally, she expands on the construct of the wild mother as supporting an individual's deep nature and urges not a disengagement from mother but rather to seek a '*wild and wise mother*' (Pinkola Estes, 1992, pp. 172–180), as in the ancient, tribal Goddess-Mothers systems, later relegated to Godmothers by religious hierarchies.

Another thread was of the development of co-dependency in their relationships as a result of this dysfunctional mothering. They shared about being unable to see themselves, being so enmeshed in the dependant relationship that they were held captive to the role of victim, appearing unable to move away from the situation and from close contact with the abusive other/dependant other. This revealed itself in several ways such as being obsessed with the other, constant criticism and complaining about the other and trying to control everyone but themselves. There were images of attack, of inflamed red-raw stomachs and painful womb-like containers depicting a trap or a prison. During one session a member described dreaming of a row of coffins and of attempting to climb into one but finding each one closed. She expressed the continued desire to be in a coffin and shared how she had stopped herself putting a piece of bark into her image to represent one. In response another member asked what her higher self wanted or needed, and she said 'rebirth'. Intriguingly, whilst creating her image a fluffy yellow caterpillar had crawled across her work; she was gently reminded of this but seemed unable to tolerate the connection. It was as though she could only envisage staying in a dark, deathly place which was familiar and known but with no possibility of change or transformation.

> Sometimes, the raw, vast, spacious truth can be too much, and we long to return to the status quo where we can forget again. Even if it feels claustrophobic and limited, we decide that it is preferable to such groundless, naked exposure.
>
> *(Matt Licata, 2017, p. 176)*

The group considered: what is it like to have a mother who sees you as being in the way of her needs, a drain on her resources, a waste, an annoyance, unwanted and even as a threat? The archetype of the Death Mother who, like Medusa, is all bitterness and wrath raising its seething, serpent laden head amongst the maternal material of the group. Horror, burning, blackness and rot crept into their art work. One member's art frequently depicted strange biological cycles as if trapped between the stomach and the head. Her other images featured amoeba-like cells filled with yellow pus with a parasite-like creature inside. Reflecting upon this, the group wondered about her attempting to digest toxins from mother. Interestingly, she described only being able to eat baby food.

In the book *Belonging* (Turner, 2017), the Death Mother is never satisfied; she gorges on the inner landscape whilst also plundering, spoiling and degrading the outer. Her appetite for destruction is voracious and there is never enough. Turner relates this to the environmental crisis, describing a Death Mother culture in which the world's vital ecosystems are knowingly compromised and potentially wiped out for the mirage that is endless economic growth (Turner, 2017, pp. 34–38).

Anger and ultimately deep grief were never far from the depths of their sharing and their art-making. Clients described feeling trapped or in a perpetual loop of fatigue, depression and hopelessness. They felt as if the mother who had devoured huge swathes of their childhood still ate away at their innards leaving in them a trail of fear and a huge wake of lack and scarcity. All that was good within them was stolen for her dark feast. Her legacy to her starving, isolated children was their inability to recognise, value and trust, all that was good within themselves or others. They spoke of a mother who cannot mother and who instead sees you as a competitor or a rival, who seeks to devour, and ultimately, annihilate you.

Trust and putting down roots

A participant considered: What did love look like, feel like? How would she find it? Where would she look? She understood only of failing, and, of betrayals and abuse. The comfort of the known easily called her back to the dark, messy, cruel world of familiar neglect. At least she understood this world. What became clear to the group was that if one had never been encouraged to risk or if any risk taken had been undermined, ridiculed or condemned, then the very process that helps to free you become the very thing that you are most afraid of: A self-imposed prison.

A lack of trust towards the feminine co-existed alongside a deep rooted and desperate need to receive, to try to regain what had been lost: the warmth, the closeness, the admiring gaze, the tender touch and the soothing voice. Group members wondered what this might be like to experience and whether this could be rediscovered or awakened. Was it even possible for the wounded inner child to take such a risk, to take a step into this hereto unknown experience? What if mother (or the transition object or person) withdrew or withheld? Would this finally prove true those feelings of original unworthiness, of stupidity, lack, blame and shame? How terrifying that one could imagine further loss and estrangement! Consequently, difficulties with parenting their own children were also prevalent.

During one session we changed our planned theme. We had originally chosen the image of a spider's web, but changed it to that of a tree because members were struggling, unable to offer themselves any kindness, encouragement or self-soothing. So we thought about a tree, about roots, earthiness and nourishment and asked: "what does a tree need to grow?" Then later, we encouraged them to relate this to the self: "what do I need to grow?" This appeared to be much more achievable; one member's image is of a bush-like tree in pastel, its dark roots are shown deeply embedded in the soil and its trunk is a series of wiry, black stems (Figure 5.1).

It has a plethora of black, green and yellow leaves. It appears healthy and strong but is being buffeted by the wind, depicted as blurry, skull-like creatures on either side of the tree. She described the tree as a family tree and the green parts and the mud surrounding the roots as protection. The flashes of yellow light on the leaves, she said, were an indication that "everything is going to be alright even if only for a moment". However, the skulls and the wind were "outside influences that fly in, knock you about and leave you with a feeling of no control".

Only knowing the wound

A difficulty for the group was that of only knowing the wound, of being so familiar with the pain, the conflict and the emotional abuse that conceiving of any difference or any change felt almost impossible. Any suggestion or hint of another way

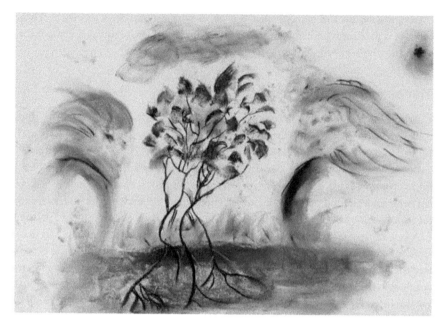

FIGURE 5.1 Tree with skulls

of being often left the client feeling further blame as if they were being challenged: "why can't you just look over here in this healthy bit?" and this led to a sense of further inadequacy: "I can't even see that healthy bit over there! What healthy bit? There is no healthy bit. I'm in a trap!"

However, what emerged in the group experience was an ability to see this contrast mirrored in nature. Yes, there was dirt, disease, decay, rot and pungency, but alongside it was growth, fragility, strength, burgeoning newness, beauty and hope. Here and there were the signs of life and renewal.

> It would take decades to realize the little acorn of my destiny needed that awful soil to grow up in.
>
> *(Turner, 2017, p. 27)*

During one particularly moving and powerful session the group ventured outside to engage in a specific exercise, one not previously practised by them. They were encouraged to become aware of something in nature and to introduce themselves to it, for instance it could be a flower, a leaf, a tree, or the sky. The members could then ask the element if it had anything to teach them or offer them, and they were to sit and listen for a response. Even sceptical members of the group found that during the exercise an unexpected, typically subtle and yet profound connection was created between themselves and their chosen element. One member was strongly drawn to a tall, lean fir tree, its almost bare trunk overshadowed by the body of the other trees with their dense canopy of branches and leaves. The sun mostly lit only the very crown of the fir tree, but there high up where the conditions were brighter pine needles grew in profusion from its upper branches. During art-making she drew the fir tree and later described finding herself in humble participation with the story of the tree. The dark, overcrowded conditions of its juvenile years had meant it had not been able to grow properly and its few remaining young branches were stubby and damaged. Standing silently next to its gnarled, black trunk she found the hardships and losses of its early years resonating deeply within her. Remembering how her young life had been marred by a particularly destructive relationship with her mother, she stood in deep communion next to it and quietly wept for her own childhood.

Figure 5.2 featured the ruddy brown, layered earth drawn in chalk pastel across an orange A3 sheet of paper. The group member had placed onto the surface of the drawing the real remains of a plant. It had only its roots intact; the stalk and main body of the plant having been removed. The roots had been uprooted from their original home and were placed instead onto the dry two-dimensional terracotta ground of the image. It is no longer a place where they can thrive, cut off from their source and suspended in space. When reflecting upon her art-making, she described being surprised at the vigorousness of her angry feelings, and during permitted feedback the group was struck at how volcanic her image looked. They expressed how the plant roots looked like they were being spewed out from the erupting molten ground, as if the half plant was being expelled like a foreign object

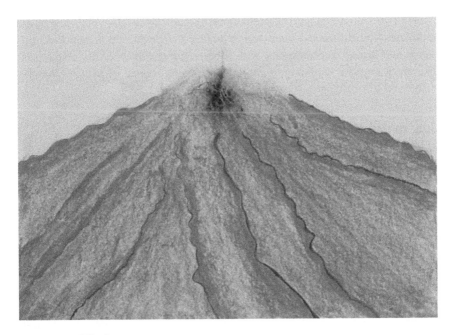

FIGURE 5.2 Weed

from the inflamed earth. The image is embodied with such strength of feeling that each time the group looked at it we saw new metaphors and meaning.

One member during an outdoor part of the session ventured to sit on a bench, and despite some initial cynicism about communicating with the elements found himself receiving insight into the trees which he observed circling around him. The trees appeared as if they knew him, like relations or ancestors, and he was able to distinguish them as male or female, old or young. He related to them as though they were real characters who had in this moment attended to him in order to support him. Although a deeply wounded and private man, he was profoundly moved and able to receive some warmth, comfort and tenderness from the experience.

At the end of the course of therapy each member of the group was invited back to a final individual review session, independent of the group except for the facilitators. During this follow-up session all of their art work from each week is reviewed, reflected upon and finally handed over to the client for their safekeeping, if they wish to have it. Within this review process group members commonly found further layers of meaning and depth to their work. Some pieces had been forgotten about and aspects of their meaning were for a moment joyfully or mournfully rekindled.

Several times during the group caterpillars and chrysalises emerged within the image making. One member had initially struggled to begin with a suggested theme and when asked if anything had resonated with her during our time outside, she tearfully expressed that an earlier encounter with a baby caterpillar had felt meaningful. She duly began a poignant and powerful image around this experience. Her caterpillar image appeared highly meaningful and she reported noticing the vulnerability of the tiny creature and its need for protection and safety.

Again she shared feelings of abandonment, rejection and neglect, reflecting upon insubstantial nurturing and premature weaning. Yet despite these ruptured, disrupted and damaged relationships with mother, group members also revealed in their work tentative explorations around burgeoning feelings of incubation, self-nurture, rebirth and transformation.

Gaia as good enough mother and learning to mother ourselves

Sometimes members reminisced about times during their lives when they had felt the freedom of being outdoors and how they had often felt soothed and comforted by nature, typically during their youth. Commonly this connection had been lost as they had grown up and become immersed in their working lives and living in the city. During their time in the group members increasingly noticed the seasons and expressed their wish that the group could run for a longer period, so that they could further delve into and understand the wheel of the year and their part within it. They also considered how the constancy of the seasons seemed to provide some stability when everything else might be changing or crumbling.

The group reflected: here was the ground holding you up, supporting you. It was not your critical mother; it was not condemning you. It simply supported you without expectation. It held you with strength and certainty, asking no favour in return. This mother will not leave or abandon you. When you go to sleep, she is there and when you wake up, she is still there. Every day of your life the ground has held you. She is steadfast, firm and enduring. She anchors and grounds you for you are her creature. Whatever you feel, whatever you have or have not done, she will not despise you. She might send a rain to wash you clean, to refresh your thirst or maybe a burst of warmth from between the clouds to warm your skin and your heart and to energise you.

The group shared: the containment of the land, the stability of the ground holds and contains us so that we feel safe enough to move, to act. The beauty of the land wakes us up; it creates awe and wonder in us. This too has a vital purpose. It is provided freely and bountifully; it is a gift, an endless supply of support, of giving to the senses and ultimately giving to the body in the form of nourishment, water and food.

Clarissa Pinkola Estes speaks of the nourished, creative life as the 'Wild Woman', the "*Rio Abajo Rio, the river beneath the river, which flows and flows and flows into our lives,*' and says that Wild Woman's river '*nurtures and grows us into beings that are like her: life givers*" (Pinkola Estes, 1992, p. 298).

Some group feedback:

"*I liked the art work everyone did and the insight from the art work*".

"*I didn't think I had anything to say but found I had loads*".

"*I had lots of fears around being in a group, but I have enjoyed it. We could relate to each other*".

"*The art therapy is different, thinking about what is inside your mind, your heart. There is lots of symbolising and I could relate to Nature more than with just the art materials*".

"*I liked going outside and bringing Nature in and talking about our week*".

"*I've loved it*".

The group also explored themes such as the container being held by the frame of the group and its boundaries, the frame of the paper and the images, the frame of the grounds and the unconditional holding of the land. Also, we explored Mother Earth as a transitional object, as holding environment, as mirror and co-therapist, and the many examples that the land gives of letting go, of following, of trust and surrender.

As I saw how members expressed their experience of mother as being to blame for their lack of nurturing, nourishment and protection, I was initially perplexed at the great depth of rage and sorrow solely directed at her. I had known in my own lineage a very gentle, forgiving, strong and nurturing mother and a similar grandmother too, now one hundred years old. My own early, personal rage had been at my father and later towards the patriarchy. I had always seen the masculine as dominating, suppressing and failing to protect, and ultimately considered many men as either a passive or active part of the 'power over paradigm'.

What I discovered in this group is that relationship with mother is a major cultural issue.

> If we as a culture have lived for countless generations waging a war of attrition against the feminine, then mothering would, I suspect, be the first thing to fail, for effective mothering requires the engagement of everything within ourselves that is heartful: intuition, bonding, holding, feeling, loving. Once these are undermined all mothering is at risk, and so all our personal experiences of Mother become tainted. In consequence here we are, the first generation in the history of humankind to be ambivalent about our great Mother the Earth, for as we fail her so for the first time she begins to fail us.
>
> *(Siddons Heginworth, 2008, personal communication)*

Decades ago Carl Jung wrote about the impact of the suppressed feminine within Christian iconography. He understood that the images we use to worship the Divine have powerful psychological impact and that the all-male deity had no equivalent feminine counterpart. Emma Jung ventured further; she expressed that when we deny the Divine feminine we also deny Nature. She believed that the masculine aspect threatened to dominate nature through intellect, science and technology. She encouraged reconciliation with nature and with its pivotal counterpart, the Divine feminine. She urged *"life is founded on the harmonious interplay of masculine and feminine forces, within the individual human being as well as without"* (Crowley, 1999, p. 83), and she described union of these opposites as one of the most vital tasks of present-day psychotherapy. Furthermore, Carl Jung revealed in his studies of the Book of Revelation his belief that after a period of destructiveness on earth Christianity would evolve and new symbols would emerge, namely the Father, the Mother and the Sun Child – the Child of Promise. Henceforth would begin a new era for humankind where the destructive masculine aspects would be harmonised through balanced restoration with the feminine.

It has taken me decades to understand and to reconcile the enormous conflict between the feminine and masculine aspects within myself and within the world, and I continue to undertake this work. Alongside this reconciliation and integration process I have continued to more fully embrace my inherent relationship with the land and to see in increasing depth how our wounds have impacted on our environment and ultimately our Earth mother. Pat McCabe, Lakota writer, artist, activist, speaker and cultural liaison has greatly inspired and supported this knowledge of both the cause and remedy of these wounds. In *The Earth Talks – Indigenous Ways of Knowing* (McCabe, 2015) Pat explains how through many centuries sacred aspects of the feminine have become forbidden, demonised and culturally despised. She describes Mother Earth as the *"heart of it all"* and reminds us of the feminine's sacred connection and synchronicity to the moon. She asks us to make a space for the feminine voice within to be heard, and highlights how the feminine speaks in a way that *"sounds so other"*. She extols focussing on the maternal lineage and the truth of who *"Woman really is, holy, life surface walker, life bringer and life bearer"* and of the urgency of realigning with this original feminine design. She describes the indigenous, ancestral maternal lineage as *"having to come forward"*, as having the power to heal women and then in turn heal the men's nation. She shares how from the Lakota perspective every living thing must play its part in the sacred hoop of life or the hoop will begin to fail, and how because humans have not upheld their part, the integrity of the hoop is now in jeopardy. Vitally, she says, women have been prevented from knowing and from living in their original design and the feminine aspect in both men and women has been denied and repressed. Ultimately, she directs that for all of us a fierce reconciliation and integration must take place around both the masculine and the feminine.

Pat describes that in this place (the British Isles) we are the keepers of a legacy, a deep relationship with Mother Earth that still stands *"like a great oak that got cut off at ground level, the root is so profound, and it reaches so deep. The root has been laying there sleeping and is waiting to be met by the top half again."* She describes how *"there are things only the heart can fulfil on behalf of the multiverse"*, and that *"the human heart is fulfilling a mission that is very precious and very necessary"* (McCabe, 2015), that despite generations of trauma its design is to be in relationship, and to love.

> The truth is you were born into beauty, as beauty for joyful life. That's the truth. We were designed for thriving life, we are perfect in that design.
>
> *(McCabe, 2015)*

In *Divine Beauty: The Invisible Embrace,* author John O'Donohue turns his complete and poetic attention to the subject of beauty. He theorises that all modern crises are essentially a crises about beauty and about the repression of beauty and says, *"the time is now ripe for beauty to surprise and liberate us"*. He extols of the beauty of the earth and our deep routed and divine connectedness to her as creatures belonging to her body, *"we are children of the earth: people to whom the outdoors is home. Nothing can separate us from the vigour and vibrancy of this inheritance"* (O'Donohue, 2003, p. 46). Beauty is the cause of community, of the arts, of harmony and of all our deepest longings, and he says, *"It unites us again with the neglected and forgotten grandeur of life"* (O'Donohue, 2003, p. 23).

To summarise what I have found through facilitating this pilot environmental arts therapy group is that it has been a powerful and restorative place for group members to express their stories of wounding, chiefly about the primary relationship with mother. It was a supported, safe and expressive space in which to be able to share their long-held feelings and to gently explore their encounter with the 'other than human', with the wild and beautiful, and with lost and forgotten aspects of themselves. I have expanded upon my understanding that to be held with trust in a group through creative, earth-based processes that encourage connection and belonging is a dynamic that fosters the revealing of the feeling self, the culturally repressed feminine self, the child self and notably the great mother self. This is the path of heart, of the hand made life and I believe it is vital, restorative work in this time of transition.

References

Crowley, V. (1999). *Jung a journey of transformation: Exploring his life and experiencing his ideas.* Great Britain: Godsfield Press.

Licata, M. (2017). *The path is everywhere: Uncovering the jewels hidden within you.* Boulder, CO: Wandering Yogi Press.

Mc Cabe, P. (2015). *The earth talks: Indigenous ways of knowing.* Dartington: Schumacher College. Retrieved from: https://youtu.be/yiDmB0ICVsM.

O'Donohue, J. (2003). *Divine beauty: The invisible embrace.* Great Britain: Bantam Books.

Pinkola Estes, C. (1992). *Women who run with the wolves: Myths and stories of the wild woman archetype.* New York: Ballantine Books.

Siddons Heginworth, I. (2008). *Environmental arts therapy and the tree of life.* Exeter: Spirit's Rest.

Turner, Toko-Pa. (2017). *Belonging: Remembering ourselves home.* Salt Spring Island, British Columbia: Her Own Room Press.

PART III

Feminine and masculine

Putting feeling first

6

MEETING THE WOUNDED FEMININE

Trauma-informed environmental arts therapy as an approach to working with physical illness

Susie Thompson

Introduction

Research is only just beginning to explore how treatment works in relation to the links between trauma and illnesses that present medically unexplainable physical symptoms, like chronic fatigue syndrome/myalgic encephalomyelitis (CFS/ME) (Frenkel et al., 2017). As a sufferer of CFS/ME, my observations and understanding about what can help clients with this illness are borne out of my own healing. I have recovered in large part due to environmental arts therapy and from learning how to work with trauma in the body. I don't claim to be cured. There is no cure for CFS/ME at present. Neither do I claim that what I've learned will help everyone who has it. However, trauma-informed environmental arts therapy has had a significant positive impact on my symptoms and energy levels and I am not alone. This chapter is the story, based on a case study inquiry, of what happened when I worked with a client who also has CFS/ME, along with some of my own experience. I hope it will lead to more people being helped in this way.

Chronic fatigue syndrome/myalgic encephalomyelitis is a debilitating physical illness characterised by extreme fatigue that is made worse by mental, emotional and physical activity and is not improved by rest. Alongside this one can expect muscle and joint pain; flu-like symptoms, sore throats and headaches; and difficulties with sleep, memory and concentration. Recovery is slow and relapses, which are common, can be triggered by stress (Institute of Medicine [IOM], 2015).

I began engaging an environmental arts therapist in 2013, whilst training to be a dramatherapist. I had previously found it difficult to express anger and to release my childhood grief, so I was inspired to find that my difficult emotions seemed to 'belong' to nature. Expressing anger felt akin to the wind ripping through the woods or my outpourings of sorrow like rain on a winter's day. I noticed that whenever I had an authentic emotional release during environmental arts therapy, my CFS/ME pain and symptoms abated for a while. I discovered CFS/ME research that showed childhood trauma and emotional suppression were common in CFS/ME sufferers (Borsini et al., 2014; Chalder and Hill, 2012). Indeed, this had been physically evidenced using Functional magnetic resonance imaging (fMRI) brain scans (Caseras et al., 2008). Emotional suppression is thought to result from the lack of safety for expressing difficult emotions (such as anger) during adverse childhood experiences. The research also showed that many CFS/ME sufferers develop behaviours to help them survive that is self-critical, people pleasing and perfectionistic (Hambrook et al., 2011). I did not find research that showed how working with emotions could impact CFS/ME, but I had found relief from my own symptoms through this. I wondered if others could be helped in a similar way.

Case study inquiry

The inquiry involved giving ten sessions of environmental arts therapy to a new female client who suffered from CFS/ME to find out if this would have a positive impact on her symptoms. Having given her informed consent, the client understood from the beginning that the therapy would be trauma-informed and have a focused aim of working towards emotional release. This may have been significant in the results.

The therapy integrated ideas developed by trauma experts such as Levine (2010) and Van der Kolk (2014) for working with the bodily symptoms of trauma sufferers. These are similar to some CFS/ME symptoms (Lindenfeld et al., 2017). I will describe the trauma techniques employed, as they became relevant during the inquiry. The environmental arts therapy drew on the natural environment using natural materials to create therapeutic art with which to interact physically. It worked with the seasons, cycles and processes of Nature and mostly took place outside in the dynamic and ever-changing natural environment. In this way, environmental arts therapy offers something significantly different to any room-based therapeutic approach. It can enable a client to engage quickly and easily, as they find themselves literally 'on a natural stage'. Though interacting with the natural world, environmental arts therapy offered an active, embodied and physically therapeutic experience. By also drawing on a mythic story associated with the land and the cycles of life, environmental arts therapy offered a creative, dramatic, symbolic and metaphorical exploration to enable the client to engage her body wisdom and her unconscious mind, as well as talking and exploring cognitively.

When I met Emma (not her real name), an intelligent and creative forty-nine-year-old, she was in a lot of pain. She had been suffering from depression for ten years and with CFS/ME for four years. She was also grieving for her husband who had died just two years before, following a short illness. Emma described her life as having been stressful and her childhood as chronically traumatic. Prior to engaging in environmental arts therapy, Emma was almost completely bedridden and desperate to provide a better life for herself and her two teenage children. She rated the severity of her symptoms at that time as being 7 out of 10 (a rating of zero would have represented having no symptoms at all).

The therapeutic landscape

It was important not to overwhelm or re-traumatise Emma and so safety and containment during the therapeutic part of the inquiry were paramount. In investigating the impact of outdoor therapy on the therapeutic relationship, Jordan and Marshall (2010) found that boundaries may be more difficult to maintain in nature than in the therapy room. Siddons-Heginworth (2008) begins and ends sessions inside a rural cabin to contain and boundary the therapy and to establish the issues and feelings the client needs to work with in nature. Emma's ninety-minute sessions also began and ended inside a summerhouse on private land adjacent to her home, which included trees, some fields and a small lake. During the middle part of our sessions, we worked outside. This session structure also took account of Emma's physical incapacity. If she had been too ill to engage outside on the land, we had the option for me to bring natural materials indoors.

As well as working outside, I used the containing structure of a mythic story for the therapy. I chose a descent myth, linked to the natural cycles and seasons of life. The myth involved a goddess losing all ability to function, then recovering and becoming more whole and, as such, provided a map for us to follow. Siddons-Heginworth (2008) asserts that goddesses in myths present an opportunity to work with the 'feminine' or feeling/being self as a balance to the more cognitive/doing 'masculine' self. This view of the masculine and feminine is not related to gender and it applies to both men and women. The theme of emotional release was present in the myth, which also included a range of characters covering a spectrum of roles, behaviour and emotions. Opportunities for Emma to work in character, rather than as herself, were important in enabling difficult emotional material to be explored at an 'aesthetic distance', where it would not be overwhelming (Landy, 1993). I had experienced this myself and it had enabled a significant moment of emotional release in my own environmental arts therapy when I had taken on the role of the 'thirteenth fairy', the one who was excluded from Sleeping Beauty's christening in the fairy tale. The woods on this occasion had provided the dramatic backdrop and the props for exploring my own exclusion from an immediate family member's wedding. The role enactment enabled me to see for the first time how I had been cast as the family scapegoat and was holding the 'shadow' for my whole family (Perera, 1981). It was a truly transformative moment when I let go of the pain of being a people pleaser, or 'good girl' and embraced the dark feminine. The dark, or wounded, feminine represents our psychological or emotional wounds (Perera, 1981), and I wanted to offer Emma the same opportunity to work therapeutically with this idea.

I decided to introduce Emma to 'The Descent of Inanna' myth. This involves the Babylonian goddess Inanna, Queen of Heaven and Earth, deciding to descend through seven gates to the underworld to pay her respects to her sister, Ereshkigal, who is grieving the loss of her husband. At each gate Inanna is required to give up one of her queenly possessions, so that when she comes before Ereshkigal she has been stripped bare. Outraged by her presence in the underworld, Ereshkigal kills Inanna and hangs her on a meat hook to rot. However, Inanna has arranged for her faithful servant, Ninshubur, to affect a rescue should she not return home after three days. This results in two tiny beings entering the underworld unseen and empathically mirroring Ereshkigal in her pain. In gratitude for their empathy she releases Inanna to them and they administer the food and water of life, which enables Inanna to be reborn.

Resourcing, as suggested by both the new and ancient literature

Trauma literature suggests identifying resources from the beginning that will enable a client to feel better when the therapy gets difficult (Taylor, 2014; Heller and LaPierre, 2012). I discovered the myth also began with this. Inanna starts her difficult journey to the underworld as a well-resourced queen, but how was Emma to begin her difficult therapeutic journey from a resourced place, given her illness? The myth begins with the line: "From the Great Above she (Inanna) opened her ear to the Great Below" (Wolkstein and Kramer, 1983, p. 52). This suggested teaching Emma to listen to her bodily self, to become aware of her internal feelings and sensations. Trauma expert Van der Kolk (2014) calls this process 'interoception', which he considers an important skill in trauma recovery. In Emma's case it helped her to understand that sometimes she experiences emotions as physical sensations or pain, something that is common in CFS/ME sufferers. Using this process, Emma was able to rate her symptoms and pain on a scale of 1 to 10 at any given moment during the therapy to know how she was doing. This was a resource we would use consistently. In the first session, I read out loud Woolley's (2002) version of the first half of the myth, while Emma laid down with her eyes closed so that she could notice if the story impacted her in any way. Emma had an unexpected physical response to the narrative (the goddess) "pours forth grain and glory to the earth" (Woolley, 2002, p. 1). Emma experienced this as if she was wearing the shining halo of the goddess. I encouraged her to imagine absorbing this "grain and glory feeling" as she called it, into her head. As she did this, her headache immediately lessened, and her muscles relaxed. This was an exciting moment, as it was the first time ever that Emma had been able to improve her symptoms instantly, indicating she had found an important resource.

Emma's physical responses to the archetypal imagery of the myth were not all positive. Hearing how Inanna descended through the seven gates into the underworld caused unpleasant physical sensations in Emma's body. When I told her how Inanna had faced her raging sister Ereshkigal, Emma's body reacted with deep pain. This physical response to Ereshkigal's anger possibly pointed to Emma being dissociated from an angry part of herself. The dissociation would likely have been a protective response to her parent's disapproval of this emotion. Emma identified with many parts of the myth, but said she was most curious about "the very brave decision Inanna took to move towards her sister's pain". Emma, however, was afraid of making that descent.

Outside in the natural world Emma explored the role of Inanna as an abundant queen through movement. Using all of her body, she opened her arms wide and described how it felt to be a queen having all of nature in service to her. When the role-play ended, Emma tracked her symptoms using interoception and found they were less painful. The role-play seemed to give her access to a healthier part of herself or to a different way of being, which is an important aspect of trauma recovery (Glass, 2006). It also produced a more positive emotional state, in which the emotions expressed were real despite the fact she was acting.

Emma was concerned that if she descended into difficult territory, no one would rescue her like Ninshubur had rescued Inanna in the myth. I encouraged Emma to find her inner Ninshubur, an internal rescuing role, as this would reduce the need for outside help (Landy, 1993). Emma identified Ninshubur as containing the quality of compassion, which she projected onto a tree whose branches touched the earth. Emma spent much of one session lying beneath her 'compassion tree', where she described feeling 'supported by the earth'. Physical encounters with nature can connect a person to qualities that they find hard to access in life (Berger and McLeod, 2006). Jordan explains that outside spaces can become therapeutic because "self and place are intrinsically intertwined with each other" (Jordan, 2015, p. 53). However, some natural environments can have a negative or dis-regulating affect and it is therefore important to check how a client feels in relation to the place they have chosen to work in. Under the compassion tree, Emma found self-compassion in being able to 'just be', stilling her worrisome internal dialogue and judging voices. These voices were possibly the internalised critical voices of her parents, which Emma used against herself (Boon et al., 2011). Emma experimented with using a calm empathic voice to soothe herself, which I had modelled for her. Gilbert (2013) suggests that through regularly summoning compassionate images from nature, compassion becomes internalised. Jordan (2015) goes further suggesting that physical engagement with the tree would have provided a positive, embodied, attachment experience, as the tree is consistent. Scannel and Gifford (2010) call this psychological bond to a place in which one feels safe 'place attachment'. This was relevant given that Emma's attachment relationship with her emotionally unavailable mother is likely to have been insecure. Over time, Emma reported that she was consistently self-soothing outside of the sessions having added the role of 'inner rescuer' to her repertoire. She said: "it's been a revelation . . . I can give myself the reassurances I need . . . I'm not just this helpless, ill person". Developing a capacity for self-soothing and self-compassion eventually enables emotions to be regulated without conscious effort (D'Agostino et al., 2017). The 'compassion tree' became another resource both as a symbolic space and as a physical place that Emma retreated to when her feelings became too intense. Emma projected safety and comfort onto trees on several occasions throughout the therapy, indicating that she was beginning to identify safe spaces within herself.

Descending to the underworld

Van der Kolk (2014) suggests helping trauma clients move towards being able to tolerate their difficult experiences and feelings. So just as Inanna gave up her possessions at each gate, Emma experimented with 'letting go' of suppressed feelings.

By working metaphorically with the seven gates enumerated in the myth, each gate enabled her emotions to be explored in a titrated, or little by little, way. This is suggested as important by Levine (2010) in order to avoid 'overwhelm', and is another area where the myth and modern theories about treating trauma coincide. The first emotion to arise for Emma was fear, which she identified as a barrier in her choice to descend.

Outside, Emma projected her fear onto a prickly stick that she found lying on the ground. The stick was so prickly that it was difficult for her to pick up, like fear, and it took her several attempts. When she finally managed to get hold of it, she was surprised and delighted to find that it felt 'light and insubstantial'. Through externalising her fear she was able to look at it in a more distanced, and therefore safer, way (Glass, 2006). By 'handling her fear' a more empowering meaning emerged as Emma realised that 'fear' had played a protective role for her against her mother's threats to commit suicide if she behaved badly as a child. While this threat of death from her primary caregiver had been shocking and traumatic for her as a child, here, as an adult, she was finally able to feel and name her anger and disgust toward her mother for this maltreatment.

Tracking the impact on Emma's symptoms through interoception and drawing on her imagery to restore balance as needed helped ensure this emotional exploration did not negatively impact her. Going back and forth between working with difficult material and resourcing is called 'pendulation' and is suggested by Levine (2010) as a way of working with traumatic material without it being overwhelming. Ogden (2009) calls this staying within the 'window of affect tolerance'. The process ended with a ritual to enable Emma to symbolically protect her inner child and develop an internal mothering role. She chose a small branch with new buds on it to represent her 'inner child' and a large piece of bark to represent 'protection', placing them together in a tree for safety. This ritual had the potential to leave Emma with a new memory of feeling protected, as neuroscience has shown that a memory can be modified and its emotional content altered through adding new information to the memory (Schiller et al., 2010).

Over the next two sessions, despite descending into difficult feelings, Emma's CFS/ME showed signs of improvement. However, at the last gate to the underworld, she divulged that her sister had recently advised Emma to "get on with your life now, because eighteen months is long enough to grieve for your husband". Emma appeared to have had no obvious emotional response to this difficult, though presumably well-intentioned, suggestion. Instead, she felt tension and pain, indicating possible suppressed emotion and an activated stress response (the autonomic nervous system, or ANS) (Van der Kolk, 2014). Interoception enabled Emma to identify that she was, in fact, experiencing 'rage'. She was surprised to realise this, yet was keen to go outside and work with it. I encouraged her to work with anger rather than rage in order to reduce the likelihood of overwhelm (Payne et al., 2015).

The intentional use of ritual enables transition from one state to another providing a containing structure for the therapeutic release of difficult emotions, and so I offered this to Emma. She decided to snap twigs from a dead tree to represent all the things she was angry about, while also expressing sorrow for the tree. This may have been sorrow for the defenceless part of herself that she projected onto the tree. She placed one twig at a time and named her anger (neglect, abandonment, loss, illness and so on). As she did so, she slowly and ritually created an anger sculpture. Interoception showed that this had elevated her ANS stress response, which she experienced as an unpleasant internal buzzing (Rothschild, 2000). Despite knowing this, she wanted to smash the sculpture to release her anger, and so I encouraged her to use her whole body and voice to achieve this. Levine (2010) suggests that by following through on 'flight' or, in this case, 'fight' actions, the body can release stuck trauma. However, having smashed the sculpture, Emma cried that her body was "weak and feeble" and that she was not strong like her sister. This may have been because she was 'under-distanced' or too close to her anger and had turned it on herself; a common response in those made to suppress anger (Woodman, 1990). I was concerned in case venting her anger had a dis-regulating affect that might cause her symptoms to worsen. However, Simpson (1997) sees symptoms as a defence against experiencing the underlying pain, suggesting that coming to terms with this pain removes the need for symptoms.

To help prevent Emma leaving the session having potentially reinforced negative ideas about herself, I offered her an imaginary strength cloak to put on. Emma played along and displayed instant changes in her physiology and attitude. She stated: "I am strong hearted even if my body is not strong, and this helps me to survive". The cloak enabled Emma to make positive meaning from the ritual and demonstrated she had easy access to her creativity, showing that well-being and good mental health was possible (Friedman, 2014).

The meat hook

In the week following the anger ritual, Emma's anxiety returned triggered by the approach of her fiftieth birthday and intense loneliness and grief for her husband. Some of Emma's grief may also have been a response to her having heard the second half of the myth. In this, Inanna, having been rescued from the meat hook, returned from the underworld on condition that she find someone to take her place there. She quickly discovered that her husband, Dumuzi, had not grieved her absence. In fury, Inanna governed that Dumuzi should take her place in the underworld for six months of the year but then on losing him, grieved his absence. I encouraged Emma to use movement to transform her physical pain and this gave her instant relief. She then retreated to the compassion tree and with the tree and I in witness and support, she cried for her husband and for herself.

I shared my observations with Emma that her grief and anxiety seemed to indicate that she was metaphorically 'on the meat hook'. Emma agreed and seemed relieved that the reality of her emotional situation had been acknowledged. However, with the admission that she was in a wretched place, Emma had crossed a threshold into a new but potentially difficult place of ambivalence (Meador, 1994). According to Perera (1981), Inanna is dynamic, fertile, and abundant; but also fierce, being both goddess of love and war. She argues that Inanna holds the opportunity for a client to become self-willed and develop an embodied and passionate life. Ereshkigal, on the other hand, is isolated, unpleasant and death dealing. As a dark goddess she is the archetypal wounded feminine. Erishkigal's underworld is not conscious but full of affect, such as despair, crisis, loss, depression, tragedy and helplessness. Perera (1981) observes that women often experience these feelings as somatic pains. However, despite her unappealing nature being monstrous, chaotic, and painful to encounter, Perera (1981) contends that Ereshkigal represents the reality that destruction and transformation are parts of the same cycle. This mirrors the natural world. Therefore, the exploration of these two opposites provides a creative opportunity to mindfully explore negative and positive effects. In so doing, I hoped Emma (the 'good girl' in control of her emotions), might learn to tolerate the ambivalence they hold (Landy, 1993), the purpose of which would be to have a regulating affect.

Encountering the wounded feminine

The next week when I saw Emma, she was so ill that she could not move from her blanketed deckchair outside her cottage, although she wanted to proceed with the session. She was consumed with physical and emotional pain, which she ascribed to over-activity on her birthday and grieving. As described earlier, over-activity can be a survival behaviour aimed at avoiding overwhelming feelings. For CFS/ME sufferers this has an intensely negative physical impact. As Emma was too ill to walk around or even engage with the natural environment, I talked her through some slow breathing exercises. I also used mindfulness and a nature visualisation to help her. This improved the pain a little, but it returned when Emma described feeling utterly alone in life and her responsibility to her children.

While visiting the bathroom mid-session Emma had an anxiety attack and on returning said that she was having "a crisis". Anxiety or panic attacks are symptoms of emotional dysregulation (Heller and LaPierre, 2012). They can be brought on by feelings such as grief, abandonment, and loss of love, all of which Emma was feeling. To restore balance and reduce her symptoms I consistently reminded her to breathe out slowly (Van der Kolk, 2014). Every time Emma spoke about her intense loneliness, the panic returned. Rumination can be a dysfunctional way of regulating difficult emotion and has been shown to negatively impact CFS/ME sufferers' recovery outcomes (Ehring and Ehlers, 2014; Cella et al., 2011). Emma's rumination clearly had an impact on the intensity of her symptoms.

The anxiety attack corresponded with the pain and chaos of an Ereshkigal encounter (Perera, 1981), located at the nadir, or lowest and worst point of the descent. As therapist, I witnessed Emma in this difficult moment and that appeared significant. By using reflective listening to echo back to Emma her distress, I was mirroring her like the two little empathic beings had mirrored Ereshkigal. Emma had been drawn to these beings and noticed this parallel with the story at the time. The ability to absorb the support being offered is potentially healing because it contradicts earlier messages of one's suffering not being taken seriously (Van der Kolk, 2014). By witnessing and soothing Emma in her distress without judgment, I hoped to show her that I could tolerate her pain and hence contradict her belief that she needed to appear 'good' to be liked. I stayed with her until the anxiety attack had finished. While it had been a difficult session, Emma later reported that after this episode she had allowed her friends to see her ill and vulnerable, instead of pretending to be well for their benefit.

The ascent

When I saw Emma the following week her appearance had the freshness of some-one whose fever had burned out. She reported having less pain and more energy and said she really understood now that she could make a difference to her symp-toms. Her unconscious process also indicated shifts. She recounted a dream follow-ing the crisis, featuring "a huge snake emerging from a manhole", while Emma calmly "went to a teashop to wait, while men on scaffolding pulled my snake out." The other people in the dream town were equally at ease with this picture. Sym-bolically, the snake is universally associated with goddesses who rule over life and death (Alban, 2010). Siddons-Heginworth describes the snake as a symbol "of the dark feminine, the wounded self" and "it sheds its skin so it can grow, just as we release layers of feeling, leaving our old selves behind" (Siddons-Heginworth, 2008, p. 41). Change happens, according to Greenberg (2011), when what was uncon-scious becomes conscious and is accepted and integrated. With these ideas in mind, Emma's dream could be interpreted as confirming her conscious acceptance of the enormity of her emotional wounds, as well as the new level of comfort she found in allowing her vulnerability to be seen by others without fear of judgment. The birth-like emergence of the snake from the belly of Mother Earth seemed to point to Emma's own re-birth from her underworld journey.

Nature's descent was ending too, with the beginning of spring, and Emma reported feeling that she had energy for the first time in years. Emma decided to metaphorically locate Inanna's realm, and this entailed finding places on the land that we had not visited before. She described these as full of "abundance, colour, and creativity". As I followed Emma, she looked completely different to the very sick woman I had met just weeks earlier. Chatting animatedly about happier times, I watched her energetically scramble through hedges and observed her delight as she found several real gateways to pass through. At each gate Emma identified either a new and positive realisation that had emerged for her from her therapy, or a hope for the future, such as a desire to create art and to be loved again.

One measure of whether the mythic journey has resulted in change is how the client copes with return, where she is confronted by familiar problems (Hartman and Zimberoff, 2005). Having finished the therapy, Emma described having made a "conscious decision to be more real with people" about how she was feeling. Instead of suppressing her emotion and 'pleasing' her judgmental in-laws, she had stood her ground with them and has been assertive with her sister. These changes in Emma's behaviour may have contributed to the improvements she was experiencing in her CFS/ME. The role of Inanna and the counter-role she had discovered in Ereshkigal had enabled Emma to understand it was acceptable, in her words "that conflicting realities can exist simultaneously". In other words, that one could be a good person and also be angry. This is integration. Integration is health (Siegal, 2010).

Conclusion

A couple of weeks after the environmental arts therapy had finished I conducted a lengthy interview with Emma. She had experienced benefits in three areas:

1   CFS/ME symptoms and energy levels

- Emma reported experiencing periods of time where she had a complete absence of pain and physical exhaustion, saying that she felt 'normal' for the first time in years.
- Her symptom improvements included a decrease in flu-like symptoms, headaches, muscle and joint pain, irritability and anxiety.
- Emma rated her symptoms as being 3 out of 10 in intensity. This is compared to 7 out of 10 prior to beginning environmental arts therapy. This decrease in symptom intensity was confirmed as lasting two weeks later, then at eight weeks, and again, two years later.

2   Behaviour and emotions

- Emma reported proactively practicing self-care and self-compassion. She continued to use the compassion tree for support.
- Her newly found assertiveness meant that she no longer needed to suppress how she was feeling in order to please those around her. This had a direct and positive impact on her symptoms.
- Emma was slowly building her physical capacity by walking around in Nature. She described being "more active and functional than I have been in a long time".
- She found "learning interoception was invaluable". Gradually increasing activity levels has been shown to improve CFS/ME (Arroll, 2014), but it is hard to gauge what is too much activity and this often results in sufferers experiencing relapses. Interoception provided a way for Emma to know at any moment whether her thoughts, activity, or emotions were too much for her to cope with. This enabled her to resource herself before continuing. She believed that this had helped build her capacity.

3   Relationship with the natural world

- Environmental arts therapy enables clients to align themselves with the natural world and its associated seasonal changes. Emma reported that it was helpful to have taken her descent during winter and to have ascended as spring came.
- Emma felt that if the therapy had not taken place outside, she would not have had access to "the power in nature". She said:

[T]he idea that you can have an emotional interface with nature is so impactful. There was something very powerful about being out amongst nature and being able to interact with it. Trees, for example, could provide protection, or become a throne, as well as being a tree. Once you've made something have a meaning, you can use it to comfort you, for example, the compassion tree.

- Emma found the myth was important too, saying "it connected us with the universality of everything in nature as well. It made me feel that I was not alone in this experience".

In comparing the experience of environmental arts therapy with the psychotherapy she had been engaged in for the previous four years, Emma said it was: "the difference between studying the territory and getting out and experiencing it. Psychotherapy is like reading a map. Environmental arts therapy is going through the terrain". In my opinion, this encapsulates the strengths of this approach. It enabled a client who had spent much of her time in bed feeling ill and ruminating to venture into the constantly changing cycles and elements of nature and physically engage with her life. In Emma's words: "exploring, feeling it, having a bodily connection to your stuff". An embodied approach aimed at releasing emotion, while not providing a total cure, had according to Emma, been "life enhancing".

Although it is not wise to generalise from a case study, it is possible that other sufferers may benefit from this type of blended therapeutic approach. Having applied all I learned here to myself (as well as to Emma), I have improved my own CFS/ME to the point where I can almost function normally. While some would say his views are controversial, Maté (2019) provides compelling research evidence for chronic stress and emotional suppression creating the underlying conditions, such as inflammation, for a multitude of modern physical illnesses. According to Maté, these include rheumatoid arthritis, multiple sclerosis, motor neuron disease, Crohn's disease, auto-immune disorders, fibromyalgia, migraine, and irritable bowel syndrome. More research is needed, but there are clearly many more opportunities for environmental arts therapists to support people with physical illnesses even beyond CFS/ME.

All over the world people are experiencing stress, emotional overload and disconnection from nature. As a planet we are in the middle of an extinction event driven by human activity (Leakey and Lewin, 1996). This is something that is within our gift to halt and yet, humanity appears to respond with emotional suppression. Perhaps these facts are too hard to look at or to imagine overcoming. Instead we have a tendency 'en masse' to busy ourselves with over-activity in order to avoid fully feeling this difficult reality. It is possible that the process described in this chapter points to the approach we need to take towards changing the fate of the planet. This means first coming into relationship with oneself through reconnection to the natural world. Then little by little acting as allies for each other in the journey, being prepared to suffer and face into the nadir. Only then may we be able to do the difficult things that are essential to create the changes needed, to heal our relationship with nature. There is hope of a return, but perhaps only after this descent. There is hard personal work to do first.

References

Alban, G.M.E. (2010). The serpent goddess Melusine: From cursed snake to Mary's shield. In Hardwick, P., and Kennedy, D. (Eds.), *The survival of myth: Innovation, singularity and alterity* (p. 23). Newcastle upon Tyne: Cambridge Scholars.

Arroll, M.A. (2014). *Chronic fatigue syndrome: What you need to know about CFS/ME*. London: Sheldon Press.

Berger, R., and McLeod, J. (2006). *Incorporating nature into therapy*. Retrieved from: http://web.a.ebscohost.com.proxy.worc.ac.uk/pafviewer?sid=45b6-a9e7-bdf77ee0716%40sessionmgr4002&vid=1&hid=4212.

Boon, S., Steele, K., and Van der Hart, O. (2011). *Coping with trauma-related dissociation: Skills training for patients and therapists*. New York: W.W. Norton & Company.

Borsini, A., Hepgul, N., Mondelli, V., Chalder, T., and Pariante, C.M. (2014). Childhood stressors in the development of fatigue syndromes: A review of the past 20 years of research. *Psychological Medicine*, 44 (09), pp. 1809–1823.

Caseras, X., Mataix-Cols, D., Rimes, K.A., Giampietro, V., Brammer, M., Zelaya, F., Chalder, T., and Godfrey, E. (2008). The neural correlates of fatigue: An exploratory imaginal fatigue provocation study in chronic fatigue syndrome. *Psychological Medicine*, 38 (7), pp. 941–951.

Cella, M., Chalder, T., and White, P.D. (2011). Does the heterogeneity of chronic fatigue syndrome moderate the response to cognitive behaviour therapy? An exploratory study. *Psychotherapy and Psychosomatics*, 80 (6), pp. 353–358.

Chalder, T., and Hill, K. (2012). Emotional processing and chronic fatigue syndrome. *Psychoanalytic Psychotherapy*, 26 (2), pp. 141–155.

D'Agostino, A., Covanti, S., Rossi Monti, M., and Starcevic, V. (2017). Reconsidering emotional dysregulation. *Psychiatric Quarterly*, 88 (4), pp. 807–825.

Ehring, T., and Ehlers, A. (2014). Does rumination mediate the relationship between emotion regulation ability and post-traumatic stress disorder? *European Journal of Psychotraumatology*. Retrieved from: http://dx.doi.org/10.3402/ejpt.v5.23547.

Estes, C.P. (1998). *Women who run with the wolves: Contacting the power of the wild woman*. London: Random House.

Frenkel, L., Swartz, L., and Bantjes, J. (2017). Chronic traumatic stress and chronic pain in the majority world: Notes towards an integrative approach. *Critical Public Health*, 28 (1), pp. 12–21.

Friedman, M.B. (2014). Creativity and psychological well-being. *Contemporary Readings in Law and Social Justice*, 6 (2), pp. 39–58.

Gilbert, P. (2013). *The compassionate mind*. London: Constable and Robinson Ltd.

Glass, J. (2006). Working toward aesthetic distance: Dramatherapy for adult victims of trauma. In Carey, L. (Ed.), *Expressive arts methods for trauma survivors* (pp. 57–71). London: Jessica Kingsley Publishers.

Greenberg, L.S. (2011). *Emotion-focused therapy*. Washington, DC: American Psychological Society.

Hambrook, D., Oldershaw, A., Rimes, K., Schmidt, U., Tchanturia, K., Treasure, J., Richards, S., and Chalder, T. (2011). Emotional expression, self-silencing, and distress tolerance in anorexia nervosa and chronic fatigue syndrome. *British Journal of Clinical Psychology*, 50 (3), pp. 310–325.

Hartman, D., and Zimberoff, D. (2005). Trauma, transitions and thriving. *Journal of Heart-Centered Therapies*, 8 (2), pp. 3–86.

Heller, L., and LaPierre, A. (2012). *Healing developmental trauma*. Berkeley, CA: North Atlantic Books.

Institute of Medicine (IOM). (2015). *Beyond myalgic encephalomyelitis/chronic fatigue syndrome: Redefining an illness* (pp. 3–9). The National Academies Press (pre publication copy). Retrieved from: www.nap.edu/catalog/19012/beyond-myalgic-encephalomyelitischronic-fatigue-syndrome-redefining-an-illness.

Jordan, M. (2015). *Nature and therapy: Understanding counselling and psychotherapy in outdoor space*. Hove: Routledge.

Jordan, M., and Marshall, H. (2010). Taking counselling and psychotherapy outside: Destruction or enrichment of the therapeutic frame? *European Journal of Psychotherapy & Counselling*, 12 (4), pp. 345–359.

Landy, R.J. (1993). *Persona and performance: The meaning of role in drama, therapy, and everyday life*. London: Jessica Kingsley Pub.

Leakey, R., and Lewin, R. (1996). *The sixth extinction: Biodiversity and its survival*. London: Orion Books.

Levine, P.A. (2010). *In an unspoken voice: How the body releases trauma and restores goodness*. Berkeley, CA: North Atlantic Books.

Lindenfeld, G., Rozelle, G., and Billiot, K. (2017). Chronic fatigue syndrome/post-traumatic stress disorder: Are they related? *Journal of Psychology and Clinical Psychiatry*, 7 (2), pp. 1–10.

Maté, G. (2019). *When the body says no: Exploring the stress-disease connection*. Bettendorf: Vermilion.

Meador, B. (1994). *Uncursing the dark: Treasures from the underworld*. Wilmette, IL: Chiron Publications.

Ogden, P. (2009). Emotion, mindfulness, and movement: Expanding the regulatory boundaries of the window of affect tolerance. In Fosher, D., Siegel, D., and Soloman, M. (Eds.), *The healing power of emotion: Affective neuroscience, development and clinical practice* (pp. 204–231). New York: W.W. Norton & Company.

Payne, P., Levine, P.A., and Crane-Godereau, M.A. (2015). Somatic experiencing: Using interoception and proprioception as core elements of trauma therapy. *Frontiers in Psychology*, 5 (93), pp. 1–18.

Perera, S.B. (1981). *Descent to the goddess: A way of initiation for women*. Toronto: Inner City Books.

Rothschild, B. (2000). *The body remembers: The psychophysiology of trauma and trauma treatment*. New York: W.W. Norton & Company.

Scannell, L., and Gifford, R. (2010). Defining place attachment: A tripartite organizing framework. *Journal of Environmental Psychology*, 30, 1–10.

Schiller, D., Monfils, M-H., Raio, C., Johnson, D.C., LeDoux, J.E., and Phelps, E.A. (2010). Preventing the return of fear in humans using reconsolidation update mechanisms. *Nature*, 463 (7277), pp. 49–53.

Siddons-Heginworth, I. (2008). *Environmental arts therapy and the tree of life*. Exeter: Spirits Rest.

Siegal, D.J. (2010). *The mindful therapist: A clinicians guide to mindsight and neural integration*. New York: W.W. Norton & Company.

Taylor, M. (2014). *Trauma therapy and clinical practice: Neuroscience, gestalt and the body*. Maidenhead: Open University Press.

Van der Kolk, B. (2014). *The body keeps the score: Mind, brain and body in the transformation of trauma*. London: Penguin Books.

Wolkstein, D., and Kramer, S.N. (1983). *Inanna, queen of heaven and earth: Her stories and hymns from Sumer*. New York: Harper & Row, p. 52.

Woodman, M. (1990). *The ravaged bridegroom: Masculinity in women*. Toronto: Inner City Books.

Woolley, G. (2002). *Inanna*. Unpublished poem. Thompson, S. (Ed.). (2014). p. 1

7

THE WOOD BETWEEN
THE WORLDS

Encountering the wounded healer in environmental arts therapy

William Secretan

Introduction

Evoking the mythological image of the centaur Chiron, Carl Gustav Jung (1956) was the first modern thinker to acknowledge the woundedness that exists in the heart of most healers. Jung regarded the clinician's own experience of personal therapy as the most important tool at the physician's disposal, observing that it is this reckoning with one's own wounds that allows the therapist to safely enter into the woundedness of the client. Further to this, as we begin to understand more of our own wounds we may begin to better understand the wounds that we inflict upon our planet and our part in the ecological crisis of our time.

In this chapter I explore my experience some years ago of being a client in environmental arts therapy. It is a window into what is normally a very private journey – a ritual journey of healing and recovery. The chapter illuminates a period at the beginning of my career as a therapist, in which I was seeking to better under-stand myself as both a man and a therapist and attempting to reconcile the seem-ingly contradictory notions of strength and vulnerability. As such, the narrative of the chapter moves back and forth between my experience as a man in therapy and also my reflections as a therapist making sense of what happened.

I had asked the environmental arts therapist that I was working with to support me in a series of sessions that would act as a male rite of passage. We both shared a notion of 'men's work' and due to our already solid relationship and familiarity with the method, my therapist and I were able to work at a depth that allowed for positive risk-taking, including physical touch, bodywork and role work. We were familiar with each other's practice and had a clear sense of the kind of work we were contracting to do which allowed for a fluidity of boundary. Environmental arts therapy can of course work at much gentler levels, with simple art-making and sharing if necessary, but because of its inherent relationship with wildness it lent itself greatly to the kind of process that I wanted to engage in.

My training as a therapist has been in wilderness therapy and dramatherapy and since qualifying as an environmental arts therapist I have also trained in psychodrama psychotherapy. Each of these modalities influences the way in which I think about and conceptualise environmental arts therapy. This chapter will not, however, be too deeply theoretical, as I seek to give a more human and accessible account of environmental arts therapy through the lens of my experience as a client. My inquiry is autoethnographic and reflexive. This transparent and self-disclosing methodology is congruent with a therapeutic practice that seeks greater authenticity in both the human and environmental encounter and is always attempting to move towards the place of greatest feeling. Guiding the reader through my experience I will show how I used environmental arts therapy as a profound and deeply effective method of exploration and change.

According to Ellis "autoethnography does not proceed linearly" (Ellis, 2004, p. 119). It is a systematic back and forth between past and present, inner and outer, thought and feeling, self and other. Ellis describes autoethnography as being like entering into "the woods without a compass" (Ellis, 2004, p. 120). So too do we enter into therapy, in the pursuit of healing, without knowledge of where the path will lead us, but trusting that the process itself will hold us in our search for truth, however exposing that inquiry may be. It is often the case that in therapy some healing comes from the growing sense that the trials we have borne as individuals are also universal human endeavours – the wounds of love and loss, sorrow and grief are both personal and existential.

Entering the theatre of the wilderness

Joseph Campbell (2012) writes that the first step on the hero's journey is the call to adventure in which, breaking away from the normal world, the protagonist is compelled to venture forth into the unknown – into the unchartered interior of the deep forest. This is analogous with crossing the threshold into the ritual arena.

Arriving on site each week, my therapist and I would walk down the muddy track towards a motorway overpass that led into the forest. As we walked, we would begin to talk. Crossing the motorway I felt like I was in another world high above the zooming traffic below. The overpass stretched across a canyon, bridging two cliff faces. At the bottom of the steep chasm, the motorway stretched out like treacherous white-water rapids speeding away beneath our feet. The bridge connected the outer world of normality to the inner world of the woods where our work was to be done.

Pearson (2013), a drama therapist, evokes the in-between world of evening when she describes how the descending sun marked a time and place, set aside by ancient peoples, to come together in ceremony. She explains that the process of getting a therapy session underway requires a similar psychological shift of light, space and time. The warm-up, or bridge-in, to each of my therapy sessions helped me to separate from everyday reality and brought me into the therapy space. This is comparable with the rituals of separation preceding many rites of passage ceremonies the world over. Turner describes this phase of transition as the "betwixt and between"

(Turner, 1967, p. 93), whereby initiates shift from their normal identities and familiar worlds and enter a liminal space where inner change can take place. Hougham (2006) uses the image of twilight to evoke a feeling of the 'space between'. This is the place where light plays tricks on our vision and shadowy figures move all around us. Our minds try to make sense of ghostly shapes, strange movements in the corners of our eyes and disembodied noises. This is the place, writes Hougham (2006), of Hermes the soul guide, who is waiting to carry us from one world to another. As I crossed the bridge I would begin to sense this twilight realm and feel the presence of something 'other'. I always knew that I was on the threshold between something inner and outer, here and there, light and dark. Like a neophyte being guided by the elders into the ancestral initiation grounds, each week I crossed the bridge, with my therapist as my guide, and entered the forest of symbols.

Once in the woods, the white-water torrent of speeding motorway cars was no longer audible, and we walked through quiet glades of young deciduous woodland steeply descending into the valley beneath us. These magical woods were the cusp-like realm between the Wardrobe and Narnia. They acted as a filter cleansing us of the noise and carbon dioxide from the road and maintaining the womb-like sanctity of the gully below.

The descent is an important image in ritual and mythology throughout the world. Whether in the Greek tale of Hades' abduction of Persephone or the Mesopotamian story of the Descent of Ishtar, descent, as a symbol of transformation, is universal. Shaw (2003) uses the story of Dante's Inferno as a metaphor for the therapeutic journey, in which the therapist, represented by Virgil, descends into hell with Dante. Shaw asserts that as therapists we must be willing to descend into the shadows with our clients, passing right over the devil's back, before we can find reconciliation. As therapists we must be willing to descend into the depths of our own experiences too before we can possibly expect our clients to do the same.

Show me the love between you and your father

The blackthorn trees were covered in white blossom like a dusting of snow all over the hedgerows. "Blackthorn is known as the crown of thorns," my therapist told me, "it tells us of the difficult tasks that must be faced." He talked about this time of year as an encounter with shadow, before the fullness of spring could be enjoyed.

We had already talked in depth about my father, a violent alcoholic, abusive and neglectful, who had often taken out his rage on me, and who committed suicide when I was nine years old. I had grappled in our conversations with whether or not I should feel anger towards my father. In truth, it was often difficult for me to feel anything tangible at all about either the violence or his death. I had previously made attempts to locate the anger that I believed I ought to feel, but on this occasion I desperately wanted to focus on the part of him that was not a monster. He was a father that I loved intensely and there were aspects of his personality that I mourned and wished I could inherit, despite all the parts I wanted to deny.

Like so many clients with childhood trauma, I found myself being constantly pulled back and forth between black and white ideas of what was 'good' and what was 'bad', when the reality was that things just weren't that clear-cut. The phenomenon of 'splitting', the polarisation of the client's experience into black or white, is commonplace in therapy. Object relations theory helps us to understand how this originates in the infant's inability to reconcile the opposites of the 'good object' parent, who is responsive and available, versus the 'bad object' parent, who is unavailable. When therapy threatens the idealised image of the good parent, clients often become defended and shut down. Despite my impulse to polarise my experiences, my therapy sessions helped me to explore these splits creatively, in a way that did not feel too overwhelming. As the reader will discover, environmental arts therapy is abundant with practical methods that allow us to sensitively and elegantly externalise these splits, so they can be worked with without being too threatening to the client's internal world.

"He was charismatic," I told my therapist,

> creative, magical and wild. He could talk to anyone, particularly those who were sick or poor . . . Dad was always making something, a piece of furniture, a sculpture, a watercolour painting – he could turn his hands to anything. He was the type of man that always had string in his pockets, ready to fashion a toy from bits of found things. These were the things I loved about him. . . .

I stopped, suddenly feeling uncertain as to whether these were my real memories, or just things that I had heard other people say about him. Were these things that I wanted him to be? Or things that I wanted to be?

Sensing depth and promise in the words I was speaking, my therapist invited me to enter more deeply into the woods and find some place, or thing, that represented the love that existed between my father and I. Straight away I noticed a hazel branch on the ground in front of me. In my mind's eye I could see the wooden swords that dad had made for me as a child. A longer branch for the blade and a shorter piece for the hand-guard, bound with string from his pocket. He would make shields too, and bows and arrows, and I had run wild in the woods of Camelot and Narnia.

I had not noticed where I was standing but my therapist had, and he pointed upwards to the trees that surrounded us. "Alder trees are sacred to Bran and Branwyn," he told me "they represent the sacrifice of the masculine on behalf of the feminine." I stood under this great alder with my sword in my hand, the bark peeling from the blade like skin from a snake's back. I tried to conjure my father into presence, picturing him in front of me, desperately trying to transmute the fragile branches in my hand into some kind of portal through which I might feel my father. He was distant, ghostly, a spectral shadow, cold and unreachable.

I could feel the solid warmth of my therapist standing by my side and tentatively he spoke,

> I'm going to invite you to reach into your coat pocket Will. I want you to imagine it's the pocket of your dad's coat. You're looking for the string he always had, but you'll find my hand instead. You can hold my hand and say what you need to say to your dad.

I cautiously reached into my pocket, and there I found a hand. My eyes were tightly shut, my body frozen with inhibition, stiff with shame. I felt so embarrassed and alone. I desperately wanted my hand to relax into the palm of his and for my tears to come, but I was a statue. I let go of his hand and set to work on the forest floor, making a grave from last year's fallen leaves to lie down in – to lie down next to my father. Stretched out next to this burial mound of leaf matter, with my eyes closed but my heart open, I was finally given the ritual of mourning that had been missing all those years ago.

Jones (1996) describes the way in which rituals of mourning can be created in dramatherapy, where they have been unsatisfactory or incomplete in reality. He stresses the ritual of mourning as a crucial part of emotional development. Children are often denied full access to the rituals surrounding death, depriving them a means of expressing grief that is both socially accepted and, most critically, held for the mourner. It suddenly occurred to me, as I lay next to the burial mound of leaves, that I had never visited my father's grave.

Dad's funeral was full of pomp and ceremony including a guard of honour from the Royal Navy, but no one mentioned the depression that had caused him to take his life. A newspaper talked about the tragic loss, but failed to mention the domestic violence, alcoholism and suicide. The whole funeral was a show for the local dignitaries, void of grief or feeling, colluding instead with a distorted, partial truth rather than welcoming the fullness of what needed to be expressed. "Grief is food to the psyche . . ." writes Somé, ". . . Just as the body needs food, the psyche needs grief to maintain a healthy balance" (Somé, 1997, p. 97). Verhaagen (2010) tells us that despite higher numbers of women suffering depression, the number of women who take their own lives is vastly outnumbered by men. He suggests that this is because men do not ask for help. What madness was this? I asked myself, as I reflected on the session. Men dying because they cannot ask for help, and then at the funerals of our dead men we, too, were totally incapable of expressing our vulnerability!

The therapy moved suddenly from the 'aesthetic distance' of the serpent-sword, to the more direct encounter of role work. I acted as my nine-year-old self, first speaking to a disembodied father, but then projecting that role onto my therapist, as I held his hand pretending that it was my dad's. Throughout these sessions, we moved from 'oblique' methods where I would find natural objects or create something to project my thoughts, feelings and memories on to, towards much more direct methods where my therapist would take on the role of a symbolic force or an aspect of an actual figure from my life.

Chesner (2019) emphasises the importance of 'psychological hygiene' when working psychodramatically in the one-to-one setting. She explains that hygiene is maintained through 'role clarity' and that this acts as a safeguard for both the client and the therapist, helping each to maintain a distinctiveness of individual experience. Despite the risks of the therapist playing a real-life antagonist, my therapist and I were working at a level of relational depth that made working in this way feel safe enough to us. My therapist only ever played symbolic aspects of my father, such as his hand, or the weight of his legacy upon me. Nevertheless, the transfer-ential phenomena were inevitable in this dynamic; I had chosen my therapist, in part, because he reminded me so much of my father. Unlike the psychoanalytic notion of 'enactment', where client and therapist unconsciously enter into old role patterns through the transference and counter-transference, in environmental arts therapy, as in psychodrama and dramatherapy, the transferential phenomena is made explicit and worked with creatively through taking on roles.

Find the man you want to be

Talking to my therapist, I told him how I often felt like an observer in situations, detached or dissociated and unable to access my own feelings or to know my own mind. How often I had observed my older brother, seemingly so able to access and express his emotions, while I felt totally unable to ever discern my own. I often found myself painfully comparing myself to my brother and feeling as though I lived in his shadow, forever second best and never quite good enough. These thoughts left me feeling voiceless, disempowered and weak.

Speaking with authority and directiveness, my therapist told me to go into the woods and find the man that I wanted to be. I walked through the woodland not knowing what I was searching for. After some time though I saw a stout oak, high up on the hillside. It was surrounded by holly trees, which grew all around its base, but the oak soared above them. I climbed up through the undergrowth and there I found an old dead holly tree, stretching upwards and gripping the oak in a tight strangle hold. Over many years the limb of the holly had slowly grown around the top of the oak's trunk.

"If this oak is me," I reflected, "then these hollies are my wounds. I have survived them, grown above them, but they still tangle around my base."

"Who then is this one holly," asked my therapist, "that still clings to your neck, gripping your throat, strangling your speech?"

I felt compelled to climb the tree. I needed to see the place where the holly gripped the oak. This was no small task. The oak was a huge mature tree. Using the old dead holly, I pulled myself upwards, slowly but surely, into the oak. I was reminded of the story of the Oak King and the Holly King, two brothers that bat-tle twice a year at the turning of the seasons. I was uncomfortable with the idea that this holly represented my own brother. What was I to do? I felt the urge to rip the holly tree away from the oak, but I did not know if I would be strong enough. Despite the holly being an old dead tree, it was firmly gripping the oak and, at its base it was still rooted in the ground. Even if I did manage to unfix the holly and send it crashing to the earth, I would then be stranded, high up in the oak, too far from the ground to jump.

I returned to the ground feeling confused. I felt that the holly did indeed repre-sent my brother and I knew that in this story I would have to defeat him in order to be free. My rational self argued back at me, defending him, reminding me that he had suffered too at the same hands, but I also knew that I had to rid myself of the grip that my feelings about him had on me. I began to slowly, tenderly remove soil from around the roots of the old holly, as if I was preparing someone to have his life support switched off. I felt somber and otherworldly. As I brushed away the soil my eyes suddenly caught sight of something clean and white in the cold dark earth beneath my fingers. I slowly parted the soil to reveal two bright bones that had begun to emerge from the ground. Two rib bones, which looked like baby serpents nesting together in the crib of the earth. There was one large and one small – big brother and little brother. I gently removed the tiny siblings, placing them somewhere safe. I understood then that my brother and I would always be bonded by our shared survival. No one else could know what we had been through together. Breaking the holly's grip on the oak's throat would not take that away, but it could perhaps give me my own freedom.

I fought my way back up through the circle of holly trees surrounding the oak, my hands and arms being scratched and cut as I scaled them. I ripped and pulled at the one that gripped the oak, tearing it from the earth, wild and raging. Finally, it dawned on me that I could ask for help and, together with my therapist, I succeeded. The old dead holly came crashing to the ground and I descended safely.

As a therapist, navigating the ambivalent relationships that a client will undoubtedly have with the significant people in their lives is extremely challenging. The loyalty that I felt towards both my dad and brother was a huge obstacle to expressing any anger that I felt towards them. At times this loyalty significantly hindered my ability to get to a place of feeling. On this occasion, the incredible discovery of two baby serpents curled up under the old dead holly was an astonishing reminder of how, sometimes, nature will do some of this work for us. They became receptacles for the love and loyalty in our relationship, which also needed to be honoured. By removing the loving part of my relationship with my brother to a place of safety, I was then able to carry out the destructive act that I needed to without constraint.

Go in search of your hidden self

I stood up from the mossy log where we always started our sessions, but instead of walking forward, as I normally did, I turned into a section of the forest hitherto unexplored. This was a journey into the underworld. The valley was littered with the bones of sheep that had strayed from the flock. We were in the shadowlands, somehow quieter than the rest of the woods. Reaching a fence that stretched across the valley, blocking our way, I asked my therapist with some trepidation, "Is it private?" This is the unconscious, I thought later – of course it is private!

We climbed over the fence and walked on into an open expanse of grass and reeds, with a stream running down one side, like a veil between planes of consciousness. Across the stream I could see a narrow strip of land enclosed by the clawing limbs of straggling brittle trees. They arched over one another like the fractured ribs of a leviathan, long dead. These ribs formed a long, dark tunnel down which I was now slowly walking.

All of a sudden, I noticed how empty my mind had been, as thoughts began to creep back into my consciousness. Until that moment, my internal world had been silent. As I was slowly drawn into the tunnel, compelled by some force of intuition, spellbound and enchanted, the tunnel had enveloped me. The ground beneath my feet squelched as the mud sucked at my boots with every step. Looking down I noticed that all around me were the deep hoof-prints of some large cloven-footed beast. My heartbeat rose, all of my senses were aroused. Something had happened here, some awful writhing battle where blustering beast had bucked and brawled fighting against an unseen adversary. I knew where I was. This was the heart of the labyrinth and I was treading the Minotaur's shadow.

The Minotaur's rage is contained and unseen, hidden as it is in the depths of the labyrinth. Those who descend and witness this rage are destroyed and never return to the surface. "I don't know if this is your rage or your father's rage," said my therapist, "but I want to invite you to experience the anger that is kept contained. I will lock my arms around you so that you cannot move yours and I want you to try and fight against my grip with all your strength and all your anger."

Standing behind me, I felt my therapist's arms wrapping around my upper body like a vice, his hands locking together at my front. I began to flex my muscles, writhing against his iron grip. I roared and screamed as I tried to shake him off me, but his arms only held tighter. We collapsed to the ground sinking into the soft mud beneath us as I struggled to break free, grunting and barking as I twisted and distorted my body. Still though, his grip remained true and unyielding until I finally gave up, breathless and panting. How deeply I recognised this rage – trapped and suffocated as it was, hidden in the shadows.

As I began to consider which direction I would take next in my exploration of the woods, I kept noticing on the other side of the stream a ruined, rusting bicycle. I tried to ignore it, turning away from its buckled, broken handlebars; its contorted, crumpled axle; cables and chain, twisted, crushed and mutilated. What was this monstrosity? This crippled chariot once whole and loved now smashed to pieces. As much as I wanted to deny this image, to discard the sight of this poor, sorry bicycle, I could not look away.

"These are the remnants of a ruined childhood," I stated bluntly. "What could have done this? What could have done so much damage?"

I hauled the bike up onto my back and carried it out of the forest.

Before the beginning of this session I had felt disengaged, flat and unable to focus on anything. As Kalmanowitz and Lloyd (2005) explain, clients can often find themselves unable to reach the aesthetic moment, or engage in the process of art-making, when they are coming close to their trauma. The capacity for absorption, imagination and creative functioning becomes paralysed. Acknowledging that everyone copes with trauma in different ways, Kalmanowitz and Lloyd (2005) write that people recover most effectively when traumatic experiences are integrated into the client's belief system. What they describe is the ability to recall experiences from the unconscious into consciousness where processing and integration can take place. Jung (1968) corroborates this idea, extolling the role of image, symbol and metaphor in bridging the gap between the conscious and unconscious realms. Within action-orientated therapies, such as environmental arts therapy, dramatic techniques can be used to externalise and witness parts of the self that have remained hitherto unseen.

In the session I had journeyed into my unconscious, where I uncovered something unexpected that had to be dragged into consciousness. Jung (1968) makes an important distinction between symbol and sign, describing the function of symbol as to express a psychological fact that the conscious mind is not immediately able to grasp, in contrast to a sign which points towards something that is already, at least partially, known. I recognised the hoof-prints of the Minotaur, and with my therapist's help, I was able to follow this sign and experience my trapped rage. The bicycle, however, was a symbol of my ruined childhood that I could not recognise until I literally carried it into consciousness. As in ritual, it is through these metaphorical images that the psychic space of liminality emerges, allowing for the crossing of a threshold between consciousness and the unconscious.

Breaking through the barrier

For the first time in this series of therapy sessions, I did not want to be here. I felt irritated by the process. I had not reflected at all on my last session. I had carried that bicycle all of the way out of the woods, forced it into my car, driven it home and placed it under the window of my study. But I could not look at it.

"I feel resistant," I told my therapist, "like I'm pushing up against something."

It was April and my therapist told me that a common theme at this time was to be born but not hatched, like the eggs in the nest. "Maybe you are pushing against the shell," he said. "What's on the other side? How does the chick know that it wants to break free? It has to break free you know."

Finally, my therapist offered an invitation, "I think you should build a barrier to break through," he said.

I found a mighty gateway between two trees, like huge pillars rising up to the canopy. It was a great muddy space to work in, and I began stomping around collecting branches and placing them between the bows of the two trees. My therapist sat on the other side of the bank watching. After a short while he offered to collect some wood.

"Yes, well you could help!" I replied sarcastically, "I wouldn't want you getting cold over there!"

Branch after branch were pressed between the trees until, like a huge blockade, the gateway was closed. I still wanted to add more. I could have kept going all day, like a beaver building his dam or an eagle erecting a huge nest. On and on I went, finding ever-larger branches and crisscrossing them through the barricade, fortifying the ramparts.

"Is this more resistance?" asked my therapist, sensing that if I could use this construction to avoid doing anything else during the session, I would. "You need to ask yourself," he continued, "if you're just building to avoid what might be on the other side."

I stood in silence, feeling exposed by my therapist's question and not wanting to acknowledge the resistance that I felt.

"Can I reflect some things back to you?" he asked. "Firstly, I'm not surprised that you haven't wanted to look at the bicycle. In our last session you went in search of a part of yourself that you didn't want to see. You brought that part into consciousness, but I would have been surprised if it had remained there. This is the part of yourself that you do not want to look at. You found the ruined remnants of your childhood."

"The second thing," he continued, "is that the two trees you've chosen to build the barrier between, that you're pushing up against, are alder trees – like the tree you found in another session to meet your father under. And the final thing I want to say is that I think you're angry with me today, and I'm wondering if this is the anger that you feel towards your dad?"

I felt confronted by the realization that through my resistance I was sabotaging myself in much the same way as my father had sabotaged himself throughout his life. I wasn't really angry with my therapist, but I was angry with myself and with my dad. My self-sabotage was the awful compulsion to build a wall around me that stopped me from feeling and from being the man that I wanted to be. This was a weight I had been carrying ever since my father's death.

I told my therapist that I felt heavy, to which he replied, "I'm going to make you feel a whole lot heavier. I'm going to climb on your back so that you can feel the weight of the old man that you are carrying around with you."

My therapist pulled himself up onto my back and I slowly began to trudge through the increasingly deep mud. With each step it gripped onto my boots with a slurping wet suction. The mud was turning to bog. I sank further and further with each step, until the sludge came up to the top of my shins. The weight of this man on my back forced me downward. I collapsed. My therapist held on, gripping firmly. I struggled beneath him, getting more and more covered in mud. He held on tighter. I kept trying to push myself up onto my feet, struggling against the weight of him. Again and again I collapsed into the bog. Finally, with my last ounce of strength, I raised myself up onto my knees. Still sinking in the bog, and with my therapist clinging to my back, I fought my way back up onto my feet and escaped the sinking black mud. Staggering over to the barricade and screaming with all my might, I threw my therapist to the ground.

We were both astonished that I had got back onto my feet, but what kind of triumph was this? To collapse beneath the weight of my father's destructive legacy and then rally on? Mustering up all of my strength to rise once again, but still carrying the old man on my back, still carrying that burden. Would I continue carrying my father forever? I needed to cut away this dead weight and rid myself of this ruinous toxic pact, this hereditary illness of self-destruction and self-sabotage.

When I was nine years old and trying to come to terms with my father's suicide and what this meant for me, I used to pretend to be him. When no one would see, I would slump down to the ground and imagine the weight of alcohol and depression, which must have hung around his neck like a lead weight, dragging him down under the water, forever drowning him. I would crawl around on all fours and imagine him within me. I would groan with desperation at my inevitable ruin.

Finding rocks by the stream, I made a body for my father, and my therapist gave me his coat to wrap them up in. My therapist held a length of twisted honeysuckle vines in his hand, plaited together in a braid. I tied this umbilical cord to my chest and felt the weight of my father pulling down beneath my heart. I felt my dad – the pulling, clinging, hungry grip. All of a sudden I was transported back to that last evening with him. How I had climbed up, onto his lap, to say goodbye. How I softly kissed him, in the sign of the cross, on his forehead, cheeks and chin. How desperate I was for some response from him. He could have already been dead, so drunk and unable to move, hear or think. I remembered the solemn ritual of farewell. Yet here I was in some sort of time warp – my adult self and my nine-year-old self, inexplicably linked and still holding on to my father, still clinging to his navy-blue jumper and flannel shirt. I finally said goodbye and tore the cord from my heart. Scooping up my therapist's coat with the body of rocks enclosed in it, I carried dad back over to the stream and tipped the rocks into the water, giving him the burial at sea he had wanted but never received.

Standing back, I still had to face the barricade which towered above me. I tracked each branch and limb of that fortress with my eyes, taking in every inch of brick and mortar, every rampart, turret and battlement. Filling my lungs, I charged at my construction roaring as I went, hitting the wall of wood at full pelt with my body, shoulder barging it with all my strength. Splintering branches flew into the air, cracking and snapping all around me, as I began to scale the stockade ripping at its fabric as I went. I stamped and smashed and climbed, pulling myself up over the parapet, bombarding the barricade until the battle was won and all around me lay the wasted debris of my own resistance.

Without ritual, how do we achieve healthy psychological separation? Campbell (2012) suggests that rites of passage can offer us the structures for a facilitated transition into independence. In environmental arts therapy it is possible to take this even further, because we are able to re-enact past situations, making our own rituals of separation. Even a ninety-year-old can have a plait of ivy attached to them and then finally cut away their umbilical cord, if that is the ritual that they need.

Find your father's shadow

On the day of my final session I awoke feeling shaken. I opened my eyes from my slumber and felt inside out, exposed and completely vulnerable. I was wide open and felt like crying, like I was a little boy, tired and confused. Arriving in the woods for the last time, I still felt shaky. I was carrying with me deep feelings of inadequacy and I expressed how fearful I was of letting myself and others down. I was scared that I would disappoint my therapist too.

"Do you think that you were a disappointment to your father?" my therapist asked, acknowledging again the transference between my dad and himself. Thinking about it for a moment, I concluded that I must have been. Surely dad projected all his own self-loathing and shame onto me. In me, he saw all of his own shortcomings and he could not cope with that, so he would lash out. Like so many clients with childhood trauma, I was used to blaming myself for the actions of a perpetrator. He would not have attacked me the way he did, I thought, had I not been a source of disappointment to him. I was quick to defend my father, rationalising his actions to my therapist, citing the abusive and neglectful childhood he had survived himself.

"I'd like you to go into the woods and build something to represent your dad," said my therapist.

> I know that you loved your dad, no one's questioning that, but I think you need to put the part of him you loved aside for the time being and acknowledge this other part of him – the angry, abusive part that would always blame and attack others.

As we walked into the woods I felt angry with my therapist, frustrated with this whole process. I knew what he was going to ask me to do – build an effigy of my dad and then knock it down, attempting to get in touch with that elusive anger. I was frustrated by the predictability of my therapist's suggestion, but even more frustrated by my instinctual sense that I would fail.

After some time walking through the woodland, seeking out some hint from my surroundings as to where I needed to go, I looked up the hillside and saw the decimated remnants of a huge fallen oak. Its shattered limbs, long dead and stripped of bark, stretched down the sloping woods towards me like the scattered debris of twisted steel and shattered concrete that emanated from Ground Zero. At the epicentre of this disastrous picture was the still-standing stump of the old oak tree, whose destruction littered the earth around me. This is the place, I thought.

With the help of my therapist, I began to build, choosing three gigantic limbs from the fallen tree to try and erect a tripod over the stump of the old dead oak. Each limb must have been fifteen feet in length and we wrestled with them for some time trying to make them stand. This was a dangerous construction, twice the frame fell crashing down to the ground and causing us both to leap to safety.

Casson (2007) describes the value of using miniatures for the client to project on to, particularly when the client has been the victim of abuse. Without something physical to represent the perpetrator, the therapist cannot know what the client is picturing, and is therefore unable to assure the client's safety, leading to the risk of re-traumatisation. Without a small object to hold the role of the abuser, unbeknownst to the therapist, the imagined abuser may be towering over the client like a giant, while the client may have shrunk to the size of a three-year-old. By choosing a tiny object to project the abuser onto, the client is assuring the advantage of size and limiting the danger of the dramatisation. This kind of aesthetic distance can help the client to maintain his or her reflective function and keep a sense of perspective from the position of witness rather than being fully absorbed into the drama.

The representation I was building, however, was colossal. It is possible that, had I been working in miniature, I may have felt less overwhelmed in my frozen trauma reaction and more able to find my own feeling response to the situation. In live therapy, however, it is often the case that these moments are guided by intuition and spontaneity, and on this occasion creating a structure of enormous size felt necessary to me. I wanted to demonstrate how huge and threatening this part of my father's legacy was. Like my father, the structure was dangerous, volatile and unwieldy – with the potential to come crashing down on us at any moment. I was a little boy next to this ogre, a vulnerable child unable to protect myself.

As disturbing as it was to think of the destructive power of this grown man towering over the little boy, so disproportionately strong and powerful, I still felt pity for him. I felt the impact of abuse going back generations and saw my father as a little boy being beaten by his father. I placed a smaller tripod at the heart of the giant to represent my father's inner child, wounded and distressed, like mine. I realised though that I could not save my father's child-self, but I could put my arm around my own inner child and carry him to safety.

I rolled up the hat that I was wearing to represent myself as a little boy and placed it in the structure. Then, after contemplating how unsafe I seemed there, I tenderly picked myself up, cradled myself in my arms and carried the symbolic object to safety. Despite this ritual of salvation for my inner child, I was still faced with the more difficult challenge of the monster towering above me. I felt absolutely powerless to confront this colossus. The weight of expectation bore down upon me, crippling me. I was so meager and impotent, so totally feeble, beneath this giant of anger and violence.

"You're doing it to protect that little boy," my therapist whispered.

Looking around I found a branch lying on the ground, like a huge club or cudgel. I lifted it up into the air like Thor's giant-slaying hammer. Screaming, I brought it down upon the destructive power of my father.

Leaving the initiation grounds behind me for the last time, I still had questions in my heart about what the experience meant for me. I started this session feeling frustrated with my therapist and resistant to the suggestions he had made. He encouraged me towards the cathartic expression of my anger, but it was the anticipation of being witnessed in this release by my therapist that most profoundly confronted me with my inner sense of fragility. It was simply terrifying to express my feelings in this way and to be witnessed by another. Despite the dramatic power of the destructive act, it was in these moments that I felt most in touch with my vulnerability and most fearful of failing to live up to my therapist's expectations. I understand more now about why I was so scared of disappointing him and why it meant so very much to me. In these sessions I was searching for my strength and attempting to better understand what it meant to be both a man and a therapist. What I found was the courage to be vulnerable – to let my raw emotions rise to the surface and, most significantly, to be seen and held in that process by another man.

Conclusion

While the intention of this chapter was simply to give an account of my experience as a client in environmental arts therapy, I had of course entered into the therapeutic process with other hopes. I wanted to better understand myself in the roles of man and therapist.

Within the prevailing contemporary narratives of masculinity, the ideas of strength and vulnerability have become seemingly irreconcilable. All too often is the vulnerable and authentic expression of feeling associated with weakness, instead of being seen as a defining characteristic of inner strength. Yet, in this account of environmental arts therapy, I hope that through my transparency I have conveyed something different. Two men, fellow travellers – one young and the other old – entered into the woods together, not knowing exactly where the path would lead them or what they would find there. The older man had walked these paths before and he knew the places in the woods where his own wounds lay, and so he helped to guide the younger man towards feeling. This was an archetypal experience of initiation – one that would be recognisable in so many ancient cultures. It is through the descent into our own woundedness that we, as therapists, are able to guide the next traveller on their journey.

The archetypes are of course present in therapy of all kinds, but it is perhaps the presence of 'the other' – Nature – in environmental arts therapy, that when combined with drama, art and ritual, magnifies our awareness of these forces by so powerfully bridging the gap between consciousness and the unconscious. When we enter into the forest of symbols, we enter more deeply into our feeling, sensing selves, connecting to the feminine part of us – the *anima*. This is an antidote to a culture in which we have all, men and women alike, been taught to distrust the feminine. It is a state of disconnection from our inner feminine that stops us from mourning our losses or expressing the fullness of our feelings. It is this disconnection that causes us to build walls, both metaphorical and literal, and which can cause us to blame and attack others for the parts of ourselves that we cannot bear. It is also perhaps this disconnection from the feminine within that leads us to attack the outer feminine and feeds our destructive relationship with the planet that we call our Mother.

References

Campbell, J. (2012). *The hero with a thousand faces*. Novato, CA: New World Library.
Casson, J. (2007). Psychodrama in miniature. In Baim, C., Burmeister, J., and Maciel, M. (Eds.), *Psychodrama: Advances in theory and practice* (pp. 201–214). New York: Routledge.
Chesner, A. (2019). *One-to-one psychodrama psychotherapy: Applications and technique*. London: Routledge.
Ellis, C. (2004). *The ethnographic I: A methodological novel about autoethnography*. Walnut Creek, CA: AltaMira Press.
Hougham, R. (2006). Numinosity, symbol and ritual in the sesame approach. *The Journal of the British Association for Dramatherapists*, 28 (2), pp. 3–7.

Jones, P. (1996). *Drama as therapy: Theatre as living.* London: Routledge.

Jung, C.G. (1956). *Symbols of transformation: An analysis of the prelude to a case of schizophrenia.* New York: Princeton University Press.

Jung, C.G. (1968). *Man and his symbols.* London: Random House Inc.

Kalmanowitz, D., and Lloyd, B. (2005). Art therapy and political violence. In Kalmanowitz, D., and Lloyd, B. (Eds.), *Art therapy and political violence: With art, without illusion* (pp. 14–34). London: Routledge.

Pearson, J. (2013). Entering the world of stories. In Pearson, J., Smail, M., and Watts, P. (Eds.), *Dramatherapy with myth and fairytale: The golden stories of sesame* (pp. 41–54). London: Jessica Kingsley Publishers.

Shaw, R. (2003). *The embodied psychotherapist: The therapist's body story.* New York: Routledge.

Somé, M.P. (1997). *Ritual: Power, healing and community.* New York: Penguin.

Turner, V. (1967). *The forest of symbols: Aspects of Ndembu ritual.* London: Cornell University Press.

Verhaagen, D. (2010). *Therapy with young men: 16–24 year olds in treatment.* New York: Routledge.

8

THE TAPPING ON THE WINDOW

Environmental arts therapy and the integrated self

Auriel Eagleton

Our shadow nature: why we need environmental arts therapy

"I hate nature". These were the words of my best friend as we picked our way through brambles and long grasses, trying (futilely) to defend our sheer stockings from the grasp of clinging foliage. I've often thought back to this moment, the adolescent vehemence we expressed, the discomfort of ill-adapted clothing, the bodily shock of crossing cold rivers and thick mud, the fundamental lack of choice that fuelled our disdain.

We were thirteen years old and seeking a sense of self-determination and identity in a world still dominated by our parents. Our undefined minds were the perfect incubators for consumerist culture, our bodies a battleground to be won. On this day gender stereotyping was winning out. We were clad in delicate tights that restricted our activity, mini-skirts and impractical pumps that pinched our heels and slipped about underfoot, unsteadying us on our perilous journey through the countryside. We fought a bitter losing battle against the elements, feeling oppressed by the imposition of physical activity and nature on our bodies, heedless of the much greater threat of insidious territorialism demarcated on the natural world (including our bodies) by popular culture and its patriarchal dominance.

If we are all part of nature then it could be argued that my friend, in expressing her anger, was retroflecting (a term used in Gestalt psychotherapy for directing feelings inward towards the self). My friend was rejecting or denying her own nature, the cellular existence that she shares with the natural world.

At the time I shared her sentiments entirely; I had little love for the natural world or my own body. Bombarded by ads for feminine hygiene products and popular television idealising airbrushed female forms, I had been separated from a full experience of self. Women's bodies were like suburban garden lawns, sprayed and weeded. Bushes were kept trim and roses pumped with hormones, blooming bigger and longer (like botoxed lips and enlarged breasts) on an otherwise sterile and characterless landscape.

I begin with this image because, living in the city, when I look around I see this world unfolding around me. There are magazines on the shelves of every super-market displaying male and female bodies as objects to be consumed. I see young adults dressed and made up to accentuate some features and diminish others, like the bleached meat and plastic-wrapped vegetables decorating the aisles. There is very little space or opportunity either to be alone or to be oneself, exactly as one is, without alteration.

Healing the split: nature, motherland and belonging

When I see clients for therapy, in my small haven in the woods in the middle of North London, a recurring theme is a sense of not 'belonging'. We talk about fami-lies who never understood them, schools that felt like prisons with gang hierarchies, enforced conformity and social ostracism, work and social cultures that are oppres-sive and limiting. Often there is a sense of not knowing who one is or what one can be in the world as vitality and self-expression are suppressed in order to survive and conform. Like my teenage self and my good friend (who now is an adult woman as much in love with nature as I am), many people are suffering a disconnect from both the natural world and their natural selves, and this can result in their experi-encing a breakdown in their lives, sometimes leading to therapy.

We usually assume that a breakdown is a negative thing, something frightening and unknown, a falling apart of the self. A German word for breakdown 'zusam-menbruch' translates literally as 'breaking together'. As a psychotherapist I find that the concept of 'breaking together' perfectly describes the journeys that I share with my clients. The breaking is actually a process of becoming whole; it is the dissolu-tion of a dysfunctional (split) way of being in the world that can ultimately lead to a healthier, more integrated and more sustainable sense of self.

For people who have lived a life-wide sense of not belonging, a return to nature can be powerfully healing. Land ownership gives us the impression of owning nature, as if it can belong to us. Yet we cannot own the myriad beings frequenting a park, a garden or a farm. We ourselves are animals and belong to the natural world and when we begin to fully trust and return to this sense of belonging, it can be deeply healing. This is the profound sense of coming home to ourselves that many of us are starved of. Embracing the 'motherland' and belonging to her is healing and fulfilling and can be totally transformative.

This chapter is about that transformation; it is about the tapping on the window of our natural selves. It is the flower pushing up through concrete, the autumn leaves blown into the house, the storm that rattles and taps at the window to remind us that we too are wild. It is the re-integration of ourselves as part of the natural world and all the sensuality, vitality and awareness carried with it.

Environmental arts therapy in practice: beginnings

Other therapists ask me how I work outdoors. It is a form of practice that challenges the traditions and assumptions of psychotherapy. It also challenges our sense of control. We enter an unpredictable environment and negotiate a world in which our clients have multiple relationships, besides the one that we share with them. When we step outside we invite clients to discover their natural selves, to see, breathe, hear and touch the natural world with wonder and intimacy. The beauty in this is that, as Ian Siddons Heginworth describes in his book *Environmental Arts Therapy and the Tree of Life* (Siddons Heginworth, 2008), this happens quite naturally because our relationship with nature is innate. We are not curators of our client's experience but witnesses and sometimes, when needed, midwife or doulas to the birthing of their inherent and natural selves.

I always begin my sessions indoors. I have the good fortune of working in a lovely wood cabin in Queen's Wood, Highgate, and a privileged place to be in the middle of the city of London. This enables me to move between indoors and outdoors, tailoring my approach to the individual needs of my clients. I like to prepare clients for working outdoors, for both the potential benefits and challenges. In particular, I like to invite clients to open themselves to a full and sensory experience of the natural world. For this I use stories.

Storytelling: an entry point into the natural world and our inherent selves

Before there was the written word there were stories. Stories are part of our biological and cultural history; they shape the way that we experience and interact with the world. Storytelling reawakens our relationship with the natural world; it speaks to our heart and its deep and enduring connection to nature's cycles.

Working with nature is heart-opening; we bring all our senses into being, we find ourselves in nature and nature within us. This practice is simple but deep. It requires a gentle, more receptive form of attention to the world, one that we are not used to giving. As we offer ourselves up in this way, as we allow ourselves to travel deep into the experience of open receptivity, we revitalize our connection with nature. We rediscover that we *are* Nature.

This process is profoundly transformative. Through the revitalization of a heart-opening and inherent connection with nature, we begin to heal the splits both within the world and within ourselves. We cannot do this practice at depth without growing to love the natural world and, in doing so, we also grow to love and accept ourselves in a way we may not have previously known.

I use my voice to tell stories and through stories I introduce people to my way of working. I invite them to rediscover, feel and know their own nature. Stories are often bound up with landscape, growing from the earth, the trees, the water, the creatures and the seasons. Siddons Heginworth (2008) uses Celtic myth and metaphor, stories birthed from British landscapes. He guides us through the seasons using the Celtic Ogham tree calendar. His stories and beautiful prose bridge the gap between our lived experience and the landscapes we inhabit. In my own environmental arts therapy practice I also use these stories, guiding people through the seasons, inviting them to re-discover themselves in land and tale, to notice *their own* passing seasons or cycles with honour and acceptance. Furthermore, I have developed my own voice, my own stories and arts-based explorations.

As an introduction to working outdoors I use a story of my own; one that weaves the threads of my environmental arts therapy approach together. It is a story about solar and lunar time, our relationship to ourselves and to nature. It is a story of beginnings. The title of this chapter is derived from this story and is an entry-point to further themes that will be covered here.

A story for beginnings: *The tapping on the window*

Once, long ago, we were wise.

"What is wisdom I hear you ask?" Can it be lost?

This is a story about knowing and unknowing the self, about knowing and unknowing our real nature. It begins with the first seed, the very seed of knowing which we have forgotten.

Long ago, before there was earth, trees or sky, before there were birds, beast or man, there was an infinite emptiness. Within that emptiness everything existed; like a rainbow containing every possibility of form, like a song containing every sound, like a dream unfolding endless unimagined stories, like a sky with ever changing weather.

For time untold colours and shapes took form in the emptiness and receded back into nothingness, songs were sung, each note forgotten as the next one rang forth, dreams decorated space, weaving together shape, sound, form and feeling, lasting only so long as a cloud formation in the sky, turning and changing with the weather.

Perhaps it was only coincidence. No one knows quite why the phenomenon of light, sound, dreams and weather combined to form a seed. It was as though the eternal emptiness had always been sought to be touched by time. In that moment time began.

The seed contained a universe and within that universe was Earth. Over time, Earth grew plants and animals, each sprouting from the memories of shapes and sounds, from the infinite ocean of emptiness through which everything came into existence. Every cell of every plant and being was made up of that same light, that same emptiness, that same potential from which all began.

For a long time the manifestations of Earth danced together like an ever-changing painting. Every leaf, every insect, every animal, every drop of water, every grain of the earth spoke, sang, played and invented. Though the creatures and animals of Earth looked, smelt, felt and sounded different, each knew intrinsically that there was no real difference, each woke in the morning with a memory of the beginning, of being one in emptiness and creation. Each felt within them the entire universe, the dance of trees, the song of water, the light of the moon, the gravity of Earth. As flower met tiger, tiger became flower and flower became tiger. It was not that their forms changed, for time had set form in the birth of all things. It was that the memory of every kind of existence originated from the same emptiness and since all life was made of the same emptiness, all beings had an internal memory of every shape, sound and feeling that had ever existed in time before time.

Time passed. Generations of creatures thrived on planet Earth but slowly the beginning faded from memory. Humans created a language. They named and categorized the beings of the world. Slowly the creatures of Earth began to experience themselves as different, as separate. Slowly the five senses became the means through which the beings of the world recognized themselves and each other, the internal emptiness of form forgotten forever, the oneness of all things un-known.

All living, moving creatures on Earth entered a kind of dream-state, believing themselves to be separate from all other things in their joy and suffering, needs and desires. They worshipped the sun for the sun allowed them to see and they began to believe that only what could be seen and touched was real. They feared the night, for each night the moon sang to them of the beginning, of the oneness and emptiness that robbed them of personal identity, of the otherness of all other things that existed within them.

Only the trees and plant-life, the earth and water remembered, for they were not confused by language or culture. They danced to the moon's song each night while most creatures of Earth hid away. For while the sun demands speed and action, the moon sings of the stillness before time and the light of dreams, it is within this stillness and the unbounded potential of dreams that the oneness of all things is felt.

As humans worshipped the sun the sun grew vain, basking in glorified power. The sun decided that he should dominate all creatures on Earth. He told them to work hard, to focus on what they could see and achieve, to be active, potent and decisive, as he was. He persuaded them that day was for wakefulness and night for sleeping, that nothing of value occurred at night and that they must act swiftly in order to make best use of his precious light.

Most humans succumbed to the sun's order, they stopped listening to the moons song, they stopped hearing the moon sing within them, they stopped feeling the trees dance or the Earth's gravitational pull. They were frightened by the dark, the moon and all things unseen or unknown. They were frightened by the otherness of all things within themselves.

As a curtain was drawn between day and night, between self and other, humans thought that they were protecting their personal power and identity, but over time they ceased to feel and to know themselves. The wisdom of the moon's song was drowned out as humans busied themselves like ants, treating the natural world as a personal resource, desensitized to the pain within themselves as they cut down trees and farmed animals for profit.

Only the most sensitive souls hear the tapping on the window, the eerie call of the trees reaching into the enclosed spaces of sitting rooms and bedrooms, calling us back to the wild.

That nightmare tapping, reminiscent of horror movies, the knobbled branch reaching into the comfort of our homes at night, that is the song of the wild within us, the story of all existence, the tigers roar and the orchids bloom.

The moon still sings if we listen, just as the plants, trees, water and earth whisper the story of our beginning, reminding us that we are more than the dream of our individual lives, that within us we are dancing trees and singing water.

As we step outside, into the natural world, we step into ourselves. As we feel the wind on our faces we hear the echo of our internal storms. As we stand still among trees and listen to the song of the moon, time takes on a different rhythm, the fast pace of the sun recedes and the moon cradles us in the memory of our eternal selves, in the simultaneous emptiness and fullness of being, in the dance of all existence of which we are part.

As we step outside I invite you to rediscover, to remember the wisdom of all things, recognizing that each tree you touch, each flower and the very mud beneath your feet is a mirror of something within you, is an echo of something you have known and lived before, is an invitation to enter into the stillness of moon-time and remember yourself there.

Why storytelling?

Telling this story before moving outdoors serves six key purposes:

1   Storytelling invites the listener to slow down, to open themselves to new or different realities. It kindles the imagination and supports a temporary release from other internal and external narratives clamouring for attention. As everyday narratives recede and a space opens for listening and experiencing, time slows down and a transition from solar to lunar time can be entered.

2   Telling a story marks the transition between indoor work and outdoor work. It marks the beginning of a new journey for the client. It is a means of honouring the journey that is being embarked upon. The story is a bridge between the studio, or clinical space, to the outdoors. It speaks of the rites of passage that the outdoors can offer, when fully embraced.

3   This story is about belonging. Acquiring a sense of belonging can be transformative. In much of my therapeutic work I encounter people who have suffered from a deep lack of belonging in their birth families and wider culture. Yet we all belong to nature and an exploration and deepening of this sense of belonging is incredibly healing.

4   The story invites the client to imagine themselves into the natural world and to experience the natural world within themselves, facilitating curiosity and reciprocity; key functions of lunar time.

5   When we listen to stories we experience ourselves within them, stories can awaken our sensory perception and we want our senses to be fully alive when we work outdoors. The intimacy of sight, sound, smell and touch in the natural world awakens us to ourselves and when we are truly receptive, when we allow ourselves to truly be with nature, we discover that we are in a relationship with an animate world; that every plant, tree and rock is as alive to us as the insects at our feet and the birds and squirrels above us.

6   The story describes nature as animate. When we work outdoors it is important to offer reverence to the natural world, to recognize the trees and plants we encounter as entities and to respect them as such.

Solar and lunar time

I place great emphasis on solar and lunar time because I believe these concepts are representative of the primary struggle of contemporary culture. We have lost touch with ways of being in and experiencing the world and each other that can be deeply nurturing and restorative. Lunar time represents a way of being in the world that values a form of mindful connection and mutuality between people and also between people and nature.

There is much talk in psychotherapy literature of a culture of narcissism. I suggest that our apathy toward and disconnect from the natural world is an extreme form of narcissism, in which empathy toward the animate world is eclipsed by homocentric pathology. Yet we cannot simply decide to see nature differently, we need practice seeing, feeling and being with her again and to do so we must also begin to feel more deeply into ourselves. Environmental arts therapy seeks to facilitate this process.

I use the concepts of solar and lunar time to highlight different ways of being in the world. I define solar time as action and goal oriented. This includes our work and daily activity and the aim is to achieve, often at the expense of what is felt. I use the concept of lunar time to highlight the importance of reconnecting with ourselves, the arts, the natural world and each other. I suggest that lunar time is felt, not measured, that lunar time is a form of mindfulness that allows us to perceive ourselves and the natural world as new, fresh, ever evolving from one moment to the next, *alive*.

So often we are caught in polarized battles of 'good' and 'bad' or concepts of duality. Concepts of solar and lunar time are not a polarity; they are not necessarily good and bad. They remind us of the need for balance between internal and external focus, between masculine and feminine, between active (reaching and directed) and receptive (experiential, being with and available to) contact with the world.

The stars still shine even as the sun's light blinds us to them. Were we to disbelieve all that is invisible to us, we would insist that during the day the sky is empty. Just as the stars wait patiently to shine and be seen at night, our real nature waits patiently for us to dim the lights of our thinking and doing and to *see* and *feel* the richness and diversity of our experience, and the emptiness that underlies our ego-centered selves. Just as we cannot see the stars shining in daylight, neither do we feel the life in the natural world, the animate existence of plant, rock, air and water.

Environmental arts therapy is about reconnecting with our archetypal history and the natural world through myth and metaphor. We are creative in and with nature, and nature is both canvas and paint. Yet we must take care not to be so egocentric as to think that nature is only that, for nature is alive in and of herself, and if we listen we can begin to hear her. The art (here defined as any form of creativity, be it image, gesture, sound, poem, story . . .) is shared, it is neither yours nor mine, it is in dialogue with nature and where such dialogue with nature begins; so ends the separation that has become so harmful to us human animals.

When we guide ourselves or others towards greater receptivity to nature, both within and without ourselves, we are not teaching something new or unknown, just reconnecting with the rich inheritance that we were born with. In environmental arts therapy I learn from each and every person I work with, because everyone brings their unique feeling and nature story with them. Consequently, I grow as a person and as an environmental arts therapist with every individual that I guide through the process. Nature is not mine to define. Other people's personal nature stories are not for me to know or to give. I am witness and doula to their re-birthing of their own lunar time.

Solar and lunar are both ways of being in the world, neither right nor wrong in themselves, a balance of both is required for healthy and fulfilled living. In Table 8.1 I give some practical examples:

TABLE 8.1 Contact styles

Example	Solar time: Active contact	Lunar time: Receptive contact
Meeting someone for the first time	This form of contact is like meeting a person for the first time and saying 'what do you do?' before even saying 'hello', before being open to feeling, before discovering and learning about the other. It is objectifying, categorizing and goal- oriented. It can be the making of acquaintances for business purposes, with no real curiosity about the person. In subtler form we may make this kind of contact every day, with the waiter we see as providing a service rather than treating as a person or with the child that we try to shape in our own image	This involves being open to experiencing the other person in the present moment, allowing for an interaction to unfold without any specific motivation or intention. We notice the feelings that are generated in ourselves while in contact with this other person, having a somatic and emotional awareness of self and other. Our curiosity about the other remains open to their inconsistencies and variations. We give the other time and space to be seen and known in all their individuality. We allow the other their variety and difference, their multitude of selves in the aliveness of being without reducing them to a purpose or category. We listen.
Star gazing	This involves measuring, categorizing and observing the night sky. We may be intentionally seeking to observe a particular phenomenon, such as a shooting star, and then labelling that phenomenon. Consequently, we may withdraw in disappointment or boredom when the expected phenomenon does not arise or respond ecstatically with a sense of accomplishment when it does.	We feel the night sky and interact with it. We watch with body, heart and mind for the sky's own gestures, myths, legends, words or images to be revealed to us. We are always open to whatever experience the sky might offer us that night, honouring the animate sky; not seeking to own, reduce or define it. We listen.
Appreciating a tree	This involves an observation of the tree, its shape, foliage and colours, comparing this tree with other trees. We may consider the value of the tree for oxygen, timber or aesthetics. We name and categorize the tree, reducing the tree to an inanimate part of the landscape, with no wisdom or experience to share and no language with which it can speak to us.	We notice a tree and in doing so notice the feelings evoked within by the tree. We spend time with the tree, exploring the boundaries between oneself and the tree, allowing one to feel the life within it. We touch the tree, being curious about all the small details while remaining present to it as a whole, as animate and interactive. We allow our experience with the tree to unfold and sit with it until the process feels complete, as though a conversation is taking place in the silence. We ask ourselves the question what is this tree in me? We listen.

(*Continued*)

TABLE 8.1 (Continued)

Example	Solar time: Active contact	Lunar time: Receptive contact
Spending time in nature	This may involve running or jogging, walking in the park, reading on a park bench or gardening. We do activities outdoors because we suspect that we will feel better for it or to keep fit or because they have to be done. We aim to complete the objective (jog a certain distance, prune a certain bush) in efficient time and then withdraw.	We allow time to journey through or sit with the natural world without a fixed intention. We allow ourselves to feel, hear and sense all that is around us. We perceive the natural world as animate, having somatic awareness of oneself within the natural world, our feelings and responses in relation to trees, plants, rocks, places. We receive our relationship with things in the natural world; things we are drawn to or avoidant of. We receive our experiences without judgement, motivation or intention. We remain open and receptive to learning, to seeing and being seen, to feeling and being felt. We listen.
Art in nature	This may involve painting a tree or landscape or creating something from or in Nature only for its aesthetic or informative qualities. We label and explain our creation, reducing the creation to something that can be owned and defined.	We allow ourselves to feel and experience nature and in this state of receptivity we make contact with our creative energy, with the feelings that are evoked, with the myths and metaphors brought to life in the natural world around. We allow words, images, gestures and sounds to stream forth as we remain simultaneously open to ourselves, Nature and the dynamic relationship between the two. We respect the art as a co-creation between ourselves and the animate world. We listen.

Listening is the very essence of receptive contact. So often we are not listening, open or curious when we are doing something with a strong motivation or intended outcome. Listening is not accomplished with the ears only, it is a state of receptivity to all that there is to experience and learn from. Listening is hearing, is perceiving, is *receiving*.

When we fully listen we receive all that is 'other', both inside and outside ourselves. In this way we integrate what is within and what is without through receptivity and dialogue.

The central content of the sessions: integration and healing through twelve monthly cycles

While the beginning of the session is introduced through story and is an invitation into experience of (and with) nature, the middle is then a dance between solar and lunar time, working with the monthly tree calendar, as described in *Environmental Arts Therapy and the Tree of Life* (Siddons Heginworth, 2008). Moving through this book is a process that invites the integration of both these masculine and feminine principles; we actively seek to see, know and experience the world through the months and seasons, yet we do this through open receptivity and connection with nature and our natural selves.

Together we explore the twelve calendar months as points in a cycle. Each month offers a cycle in and of itself; each invites us to enter into and work through our own cycle of personal experience with the natural world, moving into an ever more intimate relationship with the month and season. The year with all its seasons is a larger, encompassing cycle. During the autumn and winter months we place an emphasis on the feminine, on a partial renunciation of outer world concerns and a return inward to the depths of ourselves. This could be described as a lunar-time form of descent. During the spring and summer months, we emphasize the emergence and surging of the active masculine principle. This could be described as a solar-time form of action and reaching. Together we experience the integration of the masculine and feminine principles, feeling how the masculine is both the voice and guardian of the feminine principle when we are functioning as a whole, while the feminine offers the masculine depth and intuition from which to act in and on the world.

In each month of the year's cycle, this balance is delicately explored, giving equal acknowledgement and time to the masculine and feminine principles functioning together as a whole and also apart when dominant during a particular month or season. In this way the year mirrors the diurnal cycle; the sun shines in the daytime and then following a brief transition the moon replaces the sun in the night sky. As plants and bodies of earth, as water-filled vessels of life, we grow and are directed by both the sun and the moon and we recognize that our cycles are intimately attached to both.

In my experience, working through this cycle offers a structure and contract for outdoor work with clients. It is the heart of the work; it is the process through which the relationship to nature and the self (one's own nature) is explored. It is the phase of adventure, curiosity and personal process that brings us into relationship with the seasons in such a way that deepens our awareness of and connection to the natural world.

Furthermore, as each month and passing season offers us multiple opportunities for consciously entering into and exploring the dance between masculine and feminine (solar and lunar time), the curtain between day and night, self and other, recedes. Integration is a gradual process of experience and repetition, not exact but varied, allowing different pathways of experience to form within us but all leading to the same centre. Each pathway links or reconnects disparate parts of the self in a process of re-becoming whole.

Ending: the integrated self

The ending is the completion of a cycle; a full gestalt through which self-experience and experience of (and within) the natural world is altered and deepened. The ending is a process of honouring the journey, of recalling the beginning, of revisiting key moments or transitions along the journey and of acknowledging each rebirth and each transformation that has led to an altered experience of self and nature.

Endings are new beginnings. Environmental arts therapy does not end with the passing of a year's cycle; it begins once more with an altered appreciation and capacity for the work. Environmental arts therapy ends with the honouring of the client's relationship with nature and curiosity around how they will continue this relationship. It ends by honouring the fragments of self that have been so tenderly gathered together and carrying them into a new year without rupturing or abandoning the relationship that has been so carefully tended.

In this way environmental arts therapy is perhaps not describing a circle of the seasons but a spiral that once embarked upon continues throughout life. The work of the first cycle is tenderly enclosed in the centre of the spiral, like the heart of a flower surrounded by the growth of lush scented petals that reach into the world.

Once intimacy with landscape, tree, rock, water, weather, month and season have been fully explored and experienced, once solar time and lunar time are understood, once a person is able to navigate both smoothly and 'choice-fully', then the foundation has been laid. Once they are able to bring these principles together and through this integration remain actively and receptively in contact with themselves and the natural world, then the medicine has been passed on, the experience has been transmitted and the tools for healing returned to each person as their rightful inheritance.

Of course, while this process can be deeply healing, it does not preclude further breakages. Life is circumstantial, we cannot know or predict what is coming, and we can only work with circumstance. A person who is able to hold onto and deepen their relationship with nature and their natural selves will know how to embark on healing journeys alone or in the company of others. Inevitably everyone gets lost sometimes, veers off in the wrong direction or is blown off the path by an unexpected event. When this happens, we are invited to break together once more. The role of doulas may once more be called upon to help return us to our inherent selves. However, we may find that each time this happens the process is more conscious and therefore less traumatic and brings with it further deepening, growth and understanding.

A solo journey may be interrupted and help or support sought, but, ultimately, my intention in environmental arts therapy is to support the client's personal nature relationships and stories, and enable them to recognize that this is their birth right and a powerful means of healing that is always available to them.

When love for the diversity of all things, for the diverse images, shapes, colours, textures and scents of the natural world has been fully experienced and integrated, with it comes love and acceptance of the self. When a relationship with all things, with animal, plant, rock, earth, air and water has been fully felt and integrated, we are no longer lonely. When an acceptance of changing weather, cycles and seasons has been fully experienced and integrated, we cease to struggle and resist our own cycles and passing seasons.

With this love and acceptance of self as Nature, we are no longer objectified, split or fragmented by a culture that defines and limits us. Once a sense of total acceptance and belonging with nature is experienced, we are free of the trauma histories and family narratives that bind and limit us, free of the past, free to fully *be* in the present.

Reference

Siddons Heginworth, I. (2008). *Environmental arts therapy and the tree of life*. Exeter: Spirits Rest Books.

PART IV

The cycle of the year

Working with the seasons

9

TAKING ART THERAPY OUTDOORS

A Circle of Trees

Gary Nash

Introduction

In this chapter I describe work that I have been involved in as a contributor to the taught programme of the environmental arts therapy training course and as a practitioner delivering the 'Circle of Trees' group in my private practice. The location is North London, an urban space, where I use local parks and woodland. The content of this chapter is illustrated with working examples taken from the Circle of Trees group along with my own personal process work.

One of the principles of environmental arts therapy is that it is an integrative therapy. This includes an integration of the different arts methods, techniques and sensibilities, an integration of the arts and the therapeutic relationship as experienced out of doors; and an integrative approach to understanding how the therapeutic use of the arts in nature may contribute to psychological healing and emotional well-being. In this chapter I hope to show how the arts, creativity, and well-being are connected through the body and the imagination, and also the invaluable part that metaphor plays when we work out of doors.

As an art therapist I encourage clients, students and supervisees to actively engage with the visual arts and to develop their creative arts practice. This may involve keeping an art journal through which to imagine and visualise emotions, moods, conflicts or tensions, and to record dreams. This visual and imaginative process encourages a flow of colour, shape and form to emerge as we externalise our interior world of feelings and sensations. As we do so we find metaphors to hold and externalise emotional and psychological states. Through this practice we draw upon an inner capacity to give external form to internal feelings and to experience the restorative energies stimulated by our creativity. These internal processes can help nurture and build resilience and support the processes of self-regulation and self-reflection.

In my environmental arts therapy work I encourage clients, supervisees and trainees to develop their creative arts practice and also to develop their practice of 'being in' relationship with nature. This may involve finding and accessing natural spaces, spending time there and attuning to what might occur. This might involve walking in the woods, swimming in the ponds, sitting in the shade of a tree, lying on the earth or standing in the rain. Hence we begin to cultivate a practice of being in relationship with the natural world, touching the earth and being touched by nature. As we do so we take in the healing and restorative energies naturally occurring around us.

As my practice has developed I have found that the therapeutic benefits of both imaginative and natural processes seem to centre on how we experience ourselves through our senses. Being out of doors immediately activates our sensual awareness of self – how we move, our sense of balance, what we see or notice, the feel of the air, wind and temperature on our skin. These vital experiences are described by Martin Jordan *"Nature is animated and vital – nature becomes a space that gives the therapeutic encounter a different kind of vitality and aliveness thus aiding the therapeutic process"* (Jordan, 2016, p. 66). When, in a therapy context, we frame and hold these experiences for another, we support them to become aware that the processes of imagination and intuition also come into direct contact and expression with and through the body. It is the physicality of this process that Ronen Berger describes as *"Nature awakens our senses, inviting us to be present in the moment"* (Berger, 2017, p. 179). This awakening is experienced and deepened through our interactions and art-making with natural materials and in natural spaces.

Natural spaces: the environments that we live and work in

The lay of the land

Therapeutic work with nature can happen indoors, outdoors and in the spaces between. In my experience many practitioners on the environmental arts therapy training course live and work in urban environments, towns and villages. Some have access to common land, urban parks, National Health Service (NHS) gardens or clinical green spaces. Others work in suburban woodland, the green fringes where city meets countryside. Some practitioners work in designated therapeutic woodland or are able to take their work out into rural spaces, onto moorland, working with valleys, dykes, meadows, open pastures or Lakelands offered by the British landscape.

Many therapists work with the harsh landscapes found in our towns and cities. They may include hard tarmac playgrounds, green verges, grassy common land, municipal parks, reservoirs and ponds. They may have access to the green arteries provided by industrial highways, the canals and disused railway lines, while some are restricted to hospital, hospice or prison grounds and some to rooftop gardens. Wherever we work we take the conceptual frameworks provided by our initial training in the arts therapies, we also take our knowledge and experience of how creativity and healing are facilitated through the therapeutic relationship. The training in environmental arts therapy also supports the practitioner to relocate the principles of practice when positioning them out of doors. The training combines art-making, ritual, bodywork and active imagination with the witnessing and sharing of our feeling experience when working therapeutically with and in nature.

Emotional geographies

What responses do we have when we think of 'land' or 'earth' – how do we envisage and comprehend landscape? How is it used to define or uphold ideals, ideologies or cultural and political identities? The land can be a source of national pride and a sense of belonging. Landscape can also reflect an experience of displacement and longing represented by the forced movements of populations. Our cultural journeys and kinship histories are shaped by borders and boundaries, carved out over time so that they always hold a geopolitical connection. We are located geographically and when we think about how we define our place both politically and creatively, we need the earth and our roots to define who we think we are.

> Emotional geography attempts to understand emotion as experiential and conceptual, and how it is mediated and articulated in a socio-spatial way rather than as a purely interiorised subjective mental state.
>
> *(Jordan, 2016, p. 63)*

Jordan encourages us to think of emotions as relational flows, fluxes or currents in between people and places "rather than towards things or 'objects' – thus positioning emotions 'spatially'": *"The importance of places and their symbolic importance stems from their emotional associations and the resultant feelings they inspire"* (Jordan, 2016, p. 63). This helps us to understand the experience we have of places that we visit or inhabit and also the emotional experiences that our clients may have in relation to the spaces that we work in. When using the same therapeutic outdoor spaces I find that layers of memory and association build and accumulate over time during multiple visits. When engaging therapeutically in natural settings we experience a relationship between bodily awareness, sensory affect and memory, hooking us into a personal connection to a sense of place.

The therapeutic landscape and urban spaces

The landscapes I work with in North London include four related locations rising up and out of the city just north of Archway. The land is a raised claygate bed that runs from Hampstead Heath, through Highgate village and descends again at Muswell Hill. This area has within it two designated ancient woodlands. The workshops and training courses take place in Highgate Wood and the therapy group, the Circle of Trees, takes place on ancient hornbeam coppiced land in Queen's Wood nearby.

Since 2014 I have worked alongside Ian Siddons Heginworth to develop work-shops and training courses; planning and delivering the postgraduate certificate course in environmental arts therapy. With Vanessa Jones I have jointly delivered the Introduction to environmental arts therapy course and co-facilitated the Circle of Trees. This work uses the public open spaces provided by Hampstead Heath; the busy bustle of Waterlow Park; the safe enclosure of Highgate Wood and the open, and at times golden, outdoor-studio based in Queen's Wood.

The work began when the London Art Therapy Centre was based in Archway. Here we would work in the studio and gather natural materials from the small patch of green next door. This sparse piece of land never failed to provide an abundance of materials, even in the dead of winter. During the one-day workshops we would walk up Highgate Hill and work in the beautifully cared for Waterlow Park which provided both private and wild spaces, as well as a more public arena in which the therapy training was generally welcomed and accepted by a curious public. Our working relationship with the rangers at Highgate Wood have also enabled us to set up a tent-tipi as a temporary shelter for the days that we work with the one-year course participants. This space provides privacy and safety in a well-managed woodland environment. Here the course participants experience deep therapeutic encounters with nature during their monthly pair-work.

The move to Queens Wood has enabled me to run the Circle of Trees evening group both in the Green Studio and in the enclosed community garden. In winter we can work with the cold and dark outside, as well as in the warm and dry studio nearby, open and ready to provide shelter whenever needed. Each space has some-thing different to offer and over the years of practicing and teaching in these spaces I have found constancy and reliability in them all. There seems to be an acceptance that in natural spaces like these people can come and do whatever they need for their health and wellbeing.

Structure and shelter: indoors and outdoors

> A central feature of ecological therapy is taking clients out of doors and "into nature" – working with the client outdoors but taking the indoors framework of psychotherapy with us . . . Equally, it is possible to bring the out-of-doors indoors.
>
> *(Totton, 2012, p. 264)*

The Circle of Trees group begins in the studio, indoors, using natural materials gathered earlier in the day and also gathered by group members on their way to the session. Beginning in the studio in late autumn and continuing there through the winter season, we slowly emerge in April, fully engaging with the woodland habitat during spring and summer. Whether indoors or outside, the group begins with an opening circle (Figure 9.1); here each member chooses something from the materials collected, something that resonates with them in some way. By choosing a piece of soft moss or prickly holly, a decaying piece of bark, moist green grass or

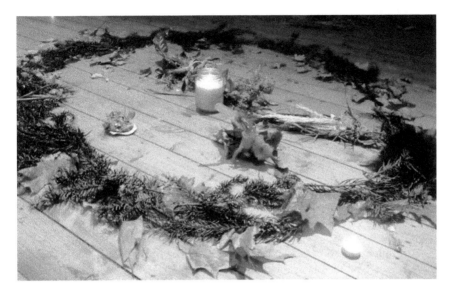

FIGURE 9.1 Natural materials in the opening circle

blossoming hawthorn, we begin to connect with the feelings that we carry into the group. We then share the feelings that we bring through the metaphors inspired by the textures, colours, appearance of (or memories associated with) the object chosen. In this way natural materials provide a metaphoric language that can help to articulate the subtle or complex feelings that we hold inside.

The opening circle is always a movement into feeling and a movement into a growing metaphoric relationship with nature. In selecting something from nature's endless palette and sharing the feeling that it evokes we introduce ourselves afresh to the group through the metaphors provided. We introduce who we are, how we are and what we are feeling as represented by the folds of lush green foliage, the spikiness of rose thorn, the softness of duck feather, the fragility of a dried out branch, the moist darkness of peat or the smell of freshly cut fungus. Using our sense of touch, smell and vision, we are stimulating the body and its memory. The opening circle also prepares the group for the work ahead, orientates new members and provides the relational dynamic that is central to any group therapy culture. Through sharing, respecting and allowing, each participant is held, heard and seen by the group. This process encourages trust building and increased levels of intimacy. Through so doing the group dynamic is engaged; this process activates the group matrix of unconscious attunement and shared empathy.

Working outdoors: the physicality of body and earth

Working out of doors provides an opportunity to touch and be touched by the world around us. Touching nature can deepen a person's "sense of his or her nature:

to feel authenticity" (Berger, 2017, p. 178). A guiding principle in the work is to slow-down, to breathe and to feel deeply into whatever is happening in this moment. When we do this often the body seems to soak up the energy, the smells and visual vitality. We are affected, subtly and gently, and if we attune our senses then we may find that this awareness grows. One's visual response may be one of awe, curiosity, interest – focusing in or taking a wide view – one's attention arrested by beauty, colour, distance or by the richness of the landscape. Our senses produce an aesthetic response through the absorption of the sights, the smells and the sensations on skin, underfoot and all around.

Working outside we begin to attune to the seasons

Autumn: The feel of the earth holding one's body; damp and firm, the smell of autumn leaves covering one's face. Noticing the warmth grow and radiate through the body, glowing under this earthy blanket. Seeing the sparkle of bright, cool October sunlight distant through the leaves under which we lay. Sinking into the musty silence, a growing stillness; a deeper sense of being held by the autumn season.

Winter: Working with frost, touching ice, the whiteness of snow; the sharp sting of the wind and the joyous aesthetic response at such a transformed world – crisp newness, fresh pathways, undisturbed and inviting. Exposed long enough and we find the increasing discomfort of cold and wetness – invigorating, exciting, tiring – a heroic brush with snow.

Spring: The lightness of feathers, working with petals, making or discovering a 'pollen path'. Finding the colour and scent of spring blossom so tantalising. The blackthorn flowers in March, holly in April, hawthorn in May, soft white flowers among the new greens. There is a heady mix of light, warmth and the scent of tree pollen as the mating begins.

Summer: The tall grasses, golden wheat and buttercups swaying in the breeze. Feeling the temperature rise, the touch of the wind, and the kiss of the sun. Feeling held and supported by the warm meadow grass, embraced by the cool shade in mid-summer. As we sink into nature so our bodies open, lightly, gently. . . . We are outside resting or moving, walking, running, breathing in through our senses.

Moving art therapy outdoors

The training in environmental arts therapy provides the arts therapist with the experience of stepping out of the studio in both group and individual contexts. Through so doing we explore the potential that natural outdoor spaces have to provide a wide range of experiences that take us gradually or suddenly into memory, feeling and bodily sensation. The therapist learns how to be with and provide a holding, containing relationship in a variable and constantly shifting space. We learn to offer an observing presence and, as in the studio when an artwork has been made and the experience is felt deeply, the therapist facilitates a space in which to reflect on this. Here we often describe and connect to a metaphoric image that can provide a verbal frame for the experience.

As we move through the one-hour time-frame of an art therapy session so we move through an analytic and therapeutic process. This involves a movement into feeling, a movement into the body, and a movement into relationship between two people and the feelings that being in relationship arouses. In art therapy we also facilitate a movement towards creativity whereby the client's visual imagination is activated along with its artistic expression. The resulting art objects or images can be affect laden, externalised emotions, fantasies, fears or memories, or dream images showing hidden thoughts or repressed feelings. In the art therapy process we then move towards a viewing/observing position where both client and therapist find a therapeutic distance from which to engage visually and imaginatively with the art piece. Here we elaborate the visual narratives and amplify the metaphors found within the form, patterns and life of the image. We deepen the possible symbolic resonance and begin to articulate some of the many meanings offered through the artwork.

When we take art therapy outdoors there is a further shift of awareness as we move in relation to what we sense and in relationship with each other, as the client leads the way towards a space in which to work. When we find the right place in nature it can feel like an arrival, discovering a space that holds meaning, something metaphoric that evokes the feeling or the essence of the material to be worked with. The space may open up, provide shelter, have the right soil or trees, some-where to climb or to dig into, somewhere exposed or a dead end, somewhere dry, arid and hard or somewhere wet, soft and boggy. Finding the space is like finding the canvas or sandtray in the therapy room, a space which can be manipulated and played with, the soil shaped and given form, the leaf litter scratched away to form an image (Figure 9.2). A space where sticks can be arranged, broken, built into towers or barricades; a place where the presence of trees, water, a meadow flowering, a hill rising, a gully deepening, can be used imaginatively and metaphorically within the client's personal narrative.

Being in nature can provide silence and solace and yet it moves also towards physicality through the senses of smell, sound, touch and vision. It can lead to handling, digging, holding, modelling, building, walking, lifting and climbing. The physical manipulation of earth, leaves, flowers, stone and wood embodies a feeling of something moving into consciousness. The sense of being in one's body or feel-ing embodied is held and subtly amplified whilst being in Nature. This awareness of the body holds a therapeutic element, as states of consciousness move from the ego-centred to a non-self-position in relation to our being held by nature. Here the thinking mind gives way to the feeling body, the defended ego begins to open and allow the feeling heart to resonate in subtle and vital ways.

I have found that nature is not just a backdrop or a stage or canvas that the client makes a creative mark or gesture on. Nature is alive, charged and interactive, and contributes to the therapeutic processes of memory, imagination and the formation

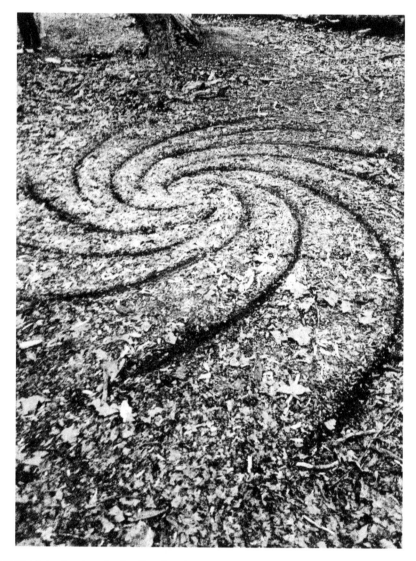

FIGURE 9.2 Land art, leaf, soil and sticks

of metaphoric associations; as well as opening the body's awareness to movements of energy and sensation. Nature enables a physical engagement and an imaginative interplay with thoughts, feelings and associations, as well as creative moments when an art piece, sound or movement occurs. Here the physicality of the therapeutic process encourages a connectedness within the client to a bodily experience of self. What can develop is an opening up and entering into a 'decentred' experience, whereby nature and mythic narratives combine and resonate internally via the imagination, and an art response emerges. Decentring is a creative therapy process and derives from drama and ritual; it is a structured movement into art-making and then a return to the real life situation with the "new possibilities of resources discovered in the art making" (Atkins and Snyder, 2018, p. 49).

Metaphors and natural materials

Fundamental to environmental arts therapy training, and a central theme running through the Circle of Trees group, is the expression of feeling through the metaphors provided by natural materials and natural spaces. The language of metaphor is essential for creative thinking and the capacity to play with objects and feelings. Metaphor allows one thing to stand for or reflect the qualities of something else and is vital if that thing is otherwise difficult to put into words. In art therapy we explore metaphor in relation to the visual narratives that emerge within the paint, charcoal or clay. Finding forms that appear, we amplify their qualities and explore their meaning or what they might communicate. We do this through the visual language of art, a language that generates multiple associations and meanings when examined through the lens of metaphor, aided by the curious 'what if' attitude of the therapist.

In environmental arts therapy this process extends to include all of nature – walking into a shady, damp and mucky pool, spending time working in the mud, feeling stuck in a toffee-like bog – what metaphoric associations might we find? Picking nettles or walking through brambles, facing a dense shoulder height wall of soft and spiky thistles; what challenges in life might they represent? Trying to shift the bulk of a fallen trunk or carrying a pile of brittle sticks; what might they represent in terms of the weight that we may be bearing in our lives? How does leaning into a mature oak or feeling the pliable support given by hazel reflect upon our need to be supported? Or how does the softness of new holly in June and the hard, prickly edges surrounding it mirror the vulnerable feelings growing inside a harsh or prickly self? Or what if we are working in the shade under hazel sensing a darkening sky overhead heavy with an approaching storm? How does making art by the dark pool resonate with looking into one's unconscious, peering into its murky depths, tipping toes and fingers into the water, touching its cool surface? Feeling one's body resonate with the cool stillness, enjoying a quiet place of reflection and then a welcoming downpour where we find ourselves soaking up the rain, or enduring a heavy heat made bearable by the protective shade of the trees. All can be experienced as metaphoric, reflecting something personal and internal.

A Circle of Trees: working with natural cycles

> The circle of trees does not just teach us about the turning year but also about the cycles of a human life as well and it is true once again that only when we are living each cycle can we truly know it.
>
> *(Siddons Heginworth, 2008, p. 179)*

Environmental arts therapy practice and theory is described by Siddons Heginworth (2008) as being grounded in the cycles of the seasons, the influence of the solar and lunar cycles, with constant reference to the particular trees defined and revealed each month. Jordan (2009) also places an emphasis on the cycles found in nature that reflect, resonate and gently amplify our own transitions and cycles. Through an attunement to the gradual changes in nature we find that our own transitions, traumas, abrupt endings, grief and losses are reflected back at us. In this way nature provides a resonance to our individual lived experience and in the context of therapy, enables us to find the words to name and share these experiences through its metaphoric language.

The term 'Circle of Trees' refers to the annual cycle of the seasons and the circle of the year, ending and beginning in tune with the larger cycles of the solar orbit. The Circle of Trees also refers to the Celtic Ogham tree calendar which places one or more specific trees in each month of the year. The Celtic year (as with other cultures that use a lunar calendar) ends in October with elder and begins in November with silver birch. The calendar follows the natural cycle and it is here that the trees drop their seeds thus beginning the cycle anew. Each tree holds metaphors that reflect a movement of energy as the seasons change in relation to the orbit of the earth:

> New beginnings of silver birch, the descent of rowan, the bridge of alder, the womb of willow, the alchemy of ash, the white track of hawthorn, the doorway of oak, the fire of holly, the dark pool of hazel, the harvest of apple, the block of ivy, the robe of elder.
>
> *(Siddons Heginworth, 2008, p. 178)*

These associations are based on an indigenous knowledge referring to trees found in European woodland and forests.

Metaphors and mythologies

I have found that as we deepen into the work there is a resonance between ourselves and the indigenous cultural associations represented by specific trees and reflected by the season we are in. As we develop a growing understanding of and attunement to nature, we find our feelings and our psychological selves mirrored and influenced by the processes experienced through nature. Another layer of metaphor also becomes available to us through the cultural mythologies associated with the sequence of trees. The intersection of human culture and nature has generated stories and produced mythic narratives which are abundant, albeit sometimes obscured. Working with these cultural stories and mythologies allows us to deepen into an experience of attunement with an older knowledge of the land, and we find that our personal and collective narratives begin to resonate. Once we begin to re-attune our senses and our imagination to the gradually changing cycles that are naturally occurring around and within us, we find that a world of deep and possibly archaic metaphors opens up to us in our therapeutic work.

The cultural mythologies that indigenous ancestors created in relation to trees and the natural landscape resonate still when we work out of doors with clients. In the Circle of Trees group, working indoors or out, we locate the tree of the month and we look, touch, smell and take in its form and substance. This will include its health properties, any cultural or historic associations, leading into the mythic tales related to these qualities. There will then be an invitation to work with the associated metaphors and to make an art-response piece (Figure 9.3). After viewing each other's work each group member is encouraged to describe their artwork, its feeling and possible meanings. The verbal description may lead to an enactment with

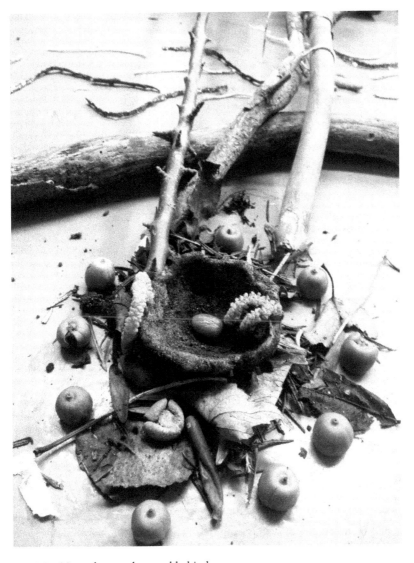

FIGURE 9.3   Natural artwork assembled indoors

the piece, or an embodied sound or movement into feeling. The use of dramatic expression through the body can take the image further as we feel into and express the energetic qualities of the response-art. Reference to a particular tree offers up metaphors for feeling, movement, energy and action which we explore and, as we do so, we find that they interconnect with a deeper archetypal experience of self, body, energy and the earth. Ritualised movement with the body, combined with expressive sound or speech through the voice, adds another therapeutic element to the work, taking the artwork further and allowing a completion of the creative gestalt cycle.

Each month is also held within a wider circle, that of the Earth spinning through its lunar and solar orbits. So as we touch into an attunement with the moment we also feel a larger energy moving everything towards cooler, darker, shorter days or warmer, lighter, shorter nights. This is a gentle, subtle, gradually moving, constantly turning energy of which we are a part.

The edges of therapeutic encounters in nature: pushing into ourselves

I first came across the work of Ian Siddons Heginworth through an article on grief, following the release of his book *Environmental Arts Therapy and the Tree of Life* in 2008. The article was published in *Resurgence* magazine (Heginworth, 2010) and made causal links between our inner psychological states and our relationship with the natural world. I was struck by a sense of my own impotence and complicity in avoiding the wider environmental concerns and ecological issues contributing to the degradation of the Earth.

This work has shown me that a lack of contact with nature reflects a lack of contact with an essential part of oneself. My experience of internal psychic loss and self-deception is reflected in my own avoidance of, and disconnection from, nature. Culturally we project onto the natural world our own internal shadow feelings of shame, fear and aggression, our own narcissistic rage and sadistic impulses, which flow freely into our natural environments, damaging all as it does so. Yet we also project onto nature our perceptions of beauty as idealised romanticism, and this alternating and contrary relationship reflects our own psychological splitting, our very own 'human nature'. It has been personally very difficult to truly open my eyes to what humanity is doing, and I wonder whether we dare rouse and waken ourselves to our own complicity. Dare we move with the creative energy that we share across species and pour that creative vitality back into our world? Is it possible?

As I work deeper with the seasonal cycle, with individuals and groups both in the studio and out of doors, I find that the increasing sensitivity and attunement to nature opens my heart. It regulates anxiety and stabilises affect and reassures me that I am embodied and in relationship with the world around me. My connectivity with nature gives me a creative vitality, resonating with the words of Mary-Jayne Rust: "*Spending time outside, whether in our back garden or in the wild, is profoundly healing, and this can be a powerful ally in helping us recover a relationship with our own nature"* (Rust, 2009, p. 45). It is this gentle but persistent energy that rises in me and in the people that I work with that becomes a creative force which flows into our lives and relationships. I find that as my contact with nature increases, so any thoughts of harming the earth feel more and more harmful to self; this conscious-ness of my inter-relationship produces a more careful tending of my own little piece of the world.

Closing the circle

Moving art therapy 'outdoors' is an ecological process. It begins as both client and therapist bring their relationship with nature into the therapy room. In this sense, the therapist holds the door open to nature's presence. Here we can acknowledge and work conceptually with nature when the symbolic language and personal con-cerns of the client refer to notions of other-than-human relationships. The practice of environmental arts therapy invites us to hold the therapy door open a little wider, to take the formal structures and symbolic processes which occur in art therapy out into the world.

During the one-year training, as in any therapy training programme, student practitioners are led into their own experience of personal process. Here we dis-cover how natural environments deeply resonate with our unique therapeutic journey. We experience how feelings and affects arise, how metaphors appear and how the active imagination can create personal associations to what is found, seen, touched and made. However large or small, these felt experiences can become deeply symbolic, standing for something hidden, dark, disturbing, shameful or repressed. In my own experience I have found that every beautiful moment holds the potential to catch or snare, to trip or uncover a dark, messy encounter with rot, death and decay, ever present in the chaotic order in all that we see and feel around us. When our exposure within nature becomes too much – too cold, too wet, too mucky, too dry, too hot, too prickly, too vast or too emotional – then we meet an edge between one's self and one's limits. Here there are opportunities and chal-lenges, a place to be tested, to push a little further, a place where we might challenge and redefine our sense of self.

In developing this work I have experienced how, when our approach as crea-tive arts therapists intersect with our knowledge of the landscape and trees that are common to the British Isles, something ancient and yet still relevant hooks us into the indigenous landscape and cultural narratives, producing an intuitive, synchro-nistic connectivity. When combined with human creativity, the physical movement and release of affect experienced in the body, plus a curiosity towards finding mean-ing in these experiences, we find a gentle and potent therapeutic process activated. When we move our arts-based practices out of doors we step into a relationship with ourselves in a fuller, more complete and complex way. Working outdoors seems to give greater space and a wider perspective through which to view our internal world of psyche, creativity, relational patterns and kinship dynamics.

References

Atkins, S., and Snyder, M. (2018). *Nature-based expressive arts therapy: Integrating the expressive arts and ecotherapy*. London and Philadelphia, PA: Jessica Kingsley Publishers.

Berger, R. (2017). Renewed by nature: Nature therapy as a framework to help people deal with crisis, trauma and loss. In Jordan, M., and Hinds, J. (Eds.), *Ecotherapy: Theory, research and practice* (pp. 177–186). London and New York: Palgrave.

Jordan, M. (2009). Back to nature. *Therapy Today*, April (pp. 28–31).

Jordan, M. (2016). Ecotherapy as psychotherapy – Towards an ecopsychotherapy. In Jordan, M., and Hinds, J. (Eds.), *Ecotherapy: Theory, research and practice* (pp. 58–69). London and New York: Palgrave.

Rust, M.J. (2009). *Why and how do therapists become ecotherapists?* In Buzzell, L., and Chalquist, C. (Eds.), *Ecotherapy: Healing with nature in mind* (pp. 37–45). San Francisco, CA: Sierra Club Books.

Siddons Heginworth, I. (2008). *Environmental arts therapy and the tree of life*. Exeter: Spirits Rest Books.

Siddons Heginworth, I. (2010). Unlocking the grief. *Resurgence*, July/August, Issue 261.

Totton, N. (2012). Nothings out of order: Towards an ecological therapy. In Rust, M.J., and Totton, N. (Eds.), *Vital signs: Psychological responses to ecological crisis* (pp. 253–264). London: Karnac Books.

10

CREATING CONNECTIONS

Introducing environmental arts therapy into London's green spaces

Simon Woodward

Introduction

Living and practicing in London and southeast England, I have offered nature-based therapeutic workshops to participants from diverse backgrounds. Developed through COATS (Community Outdoor Art Therapy Service) a collective of outdoor art therapists, this work has evolved through a synthesis of environmental arts therapy learning, conventional art therapy principles and my own connection with the natural world.

Working in urban parks and woodland one is only too aware of the tensions that exist between the needs of human beings and that of wildlife. However, these green spaces provide more than just a pleasant place to visit – they are an opportunity to reconnect with the ancient, eternal and elemental aspects of nature. The history of these public places is intimately linked to the changing relationship people have had with the natural world over the years: "Accessible greenspace, particularly in urban areas, is now becoming recognised as providing some of the fundamental needs of society, rather than just being 'nice to have'" (Natural England, 2010, p. 9).

Within an urban population, clients may well have some form of connection with nature but may not be daily and consistently immersed in it. An urban populations' engagement with nature can range from simply looking out onto a natural scene through a window to intentionally seeking out natural spaces to visit. A study by Cox, Fuller, Gaston, Hudson, and Shanahan (2017) conducted in southeast England concluded: "... *accumulatively 75% of interactions where people were actually present in nature were experienced by just 32% of the population. Indeed, people who directly experience nature regularly in any given week are clearly the exception rather than the norm*" (p. 79).

This study reflects my own experience of working in urban green spaces. Some clients' lack of direct experience of being in nature was reflected in their choice of clothes or footwear – seemingly influenced more by street fashion rather than the practicalities of being outdoors. Instinctive reactions to close contact with earth and soil varied enormously – from those that welcomed the experience to those whose anxiety inhibited direct contact. In addition, many of the clients I worked with in the COATS projects (described below) had some form of anxiety that inhibited their life choices. Just the act of turning up for an outdoor workshop away from the safe confines of familiar indoor spaces was an achievement in itself.

However, the majority of clients expressed an innate understanding that connecting with nature made them feel better. Deeper parts of our psyche are still rooted in a time when our survival depended on an intimate, felt knowledge of the natural world. Globally, our reconnection with nature on an individual and societal level is becoming even more pressing as the effects of climate change and biodiversity loss begin to be experienced as a very real threat to our health and well-being. Creating a reciprocal, respectful relationship feels a fundamental part of any attempt to connect with nature. This is not only pertinent to how we treat the environment but each other.

Working therapeutically outdoors with individuals or groups brings together these two principles – simultaneous connection with both nature and other human beings. Further, exploring the connection between inner worlds and the experience of outer natural spaces facilitates the psychic healing central to the therapeutic process. The mechanism by which this occurs is through projection: "Projection as a mechanism allows us to gain access to inner reality by using the outer world as a place where we may be able to understand our feelings more clearly" (Jordan, 2015, p. 67). Art therapy uses projection whereby the external art object can hold the feelings before they are reintegrated. The natural world offers additional opportunities for understanding ourselves through a tangible external experience using all our senses. Within environmental arts therapy this is further enriched through myths, the universal narratives that resonate with our own story and multi-layered metaphors.

Working alongside my COATS colleagues, I have borne witness to this process time and again. Consequently, our outdoor work has developed from both an instinctive understanding of the benefits of connecting with nature and evidence-based research:

> The aim of COATS is to integrate ecotherapy and art therapy concepts to provide therapeutic and social engagement that empowers participants through self-expression using natural materials and their relationship to the natural world. Our intention is to promote and integrate the mental and physical wellbeing of group participants. Engendering emotional growth through social interaction can be aided by a shared experience – through art making and engaging with nature. Additionally, the sharing of nature and artistic expression is not constricted by social or cultural identity.
>
> *(COATS, 2018)*

We drew upon a wide range of sources to create our guiding philosophy. Inspired by the national Ecominds project (Mind, 2013) we incorporated the Five Ways to Wellbeing model into our practice (Government Office for Science, 2008, p. 23). Its recommendations listed below resonate with nature-based therapy:

1   *Connect . . . With the people around you.*
2   *Be active . . . Go for a walk or run. Step outside.*
3   *Take notice . . . Be curious. Catch sight of the beautiful . . . Notice the changing seasons . . . Be aware of the world . . . Reflecting on your experiences will help you appreciate what matters to you.*
4   *Keep learning*
5   *Give . . . Join a community group. . . . Look out, as well as in. . . . Seeing yourself, and your happiness, as linked to the wider community creates connections with the people around you.*

A 2008 report created by the Centre for Well-being at the New Economics Foundation on behalf of the Foresight project highlighted the risk factors of urbanisation for future trends in mental health disorders. In addition, it states: "Growing evidence suggests that contact with the natural world is also thought to have benefits for mental health" (New Economics Foundation, 2008, p. 12). Aspects of the Five Ways, particularly noticing the changing seasons, creating community through connection and reflecting on your experiences offers parallels with environmental arts therapy principles. These have been interwoven into projects provided by COATS, offering a spectrum of ways to engage therapeutically with nature:

- Traditional myths and modern interpretations of ancient rituals
- Using metaphor that builds connections between everyday experiences of nature and psychic processes
- Direct, sensuous engagement through art-making

The challenge was to offer an accessible connection to nature and the seasonal metaphors at the heart of environmental arts therapy without taking urban clients too far out of their comfort zone. As a result, the projects were structured using a containing, directive approach, appealing to as broad a range of clients as possible – including those that may not be familiar with regularly being immersed in nature.

The format of the projects followed the framework of: check-in, grounding meditation, foraging for natural art materials, art-making and group reflection. These are usually facilitated between two hours to half a day. In the following exploration I will consider the context of a selection of COATS projects – their aims, location and participants' mental health or well-being needs and how they link to the principles of environmental arts therapy.

Consideration will be given to the communication and connection of the participants' relationship with nature and with other people.

Studio Upstairs

Between 2012 and 2015 I worked at Studio Upstairs, North London, as an art therapist and studio manager. An adult therapeutic arts community located in three centres: Bristol, South London and North London, Studio Upstairs provides: "holistic support to people who are experiencing enduring mental or emotional difficulties so that they can re-create their reasons and purpose for living, find new ways to live and experience a better quality of life" (Studio Upstairs, 2017).

I ran four seasonally themed workshops for Studio Upstairs at Springfield Park. This green space in East London has an element of wildness about it. The park offers a graduated introduction to being in nature, starting as manicured lawns and flower beds, then descending a wilder slope of woodland and tall grasses before arriving at the River Lea and Leyton marshes beyond. The park has also been designated a site of importance for nature conservation. Within the woodland I discovered a natural circular clearing in the trees. At its entrance stood a scarlet oak (one of nine species of oak in the park). It had the feel of a natural amphitheatre – light and open but at the same time hidden from view. The participants were offered a mythological theme for each of the four workshops as a starting point to their afternoon of art-making. These are listed in chronological order below.

Autumn

Out of the nine people who expressed an interest, three participated. My under-standing of the studio members is that sometimes their anxiety can inhibit them from engaging with activities that are not part of their usual routine. This was powerfully demonstrated as we walked along the River Lea to get to the park. We were all fascinated by the colourful spiders, their webs defying our expectations of where they could be feasible constructed. We all stood for a moment and gazed in silence at a particularly large web and the orb spider at its centre. The feeling of being connected through a shared experience was palpable in that moment of looking together. One member eventually said that this was the first workshop that she had ever attended and had been encouraged by my calm demeanour. However, it is my feeling that the joint attention (Isserow, 2008) elicited by the web and its potent metaphor of connection had allowed the member to verbalise her feelings.

Once we had reached Springfield Park and settled into the chosen clearing, I introduced the participants to the theme of harvest and the Celtic name for the celebration, 'Mabon'. We considered how we often don't take time to stop and think about our achievements, and that at this time of year we can celebrate our successes, the fruits of our labour. We also thought about wishes for the coming year – things that we wanted to bear fruit. As this was at the autumnal equinox, we used the metaphor of equal day and night in relation to creating balance in one's life. We reflected on the process of harvesting – the act of sorting out this from that, of cutting away what is unnecessary. Consequently, we decided to create art around letting go of something that was no longer needed.

The members were also guided through a visualisation meditation in which they imagined they were a tree drawing sustenance from their roots whilst their leaves used sunlight to produce first blossom, then fruit. During the meditation, Chloe (pseudonym) chose not to close her eyes and I wondered whether this was a form of hyper-vigilance. Luke (pseudonym) said that the meditation allowed him to really slow down and connect with the immediate natural environment.

Later, looking at Luke's face, his general demeanour genuinely appeared to be more relaxed. I felt a shift in energy throughout the entire group on completing the meditation.

The foraging of art materials and art-making merged into one process. Initially, there had been some individual anxiety about going off to look for items, so we moved as a group which seemed to ameliorate this fear. However, once the participants had left the immediate space, they quickly found their own way. Luke and Chloe migrated back and forth with their chosen items, alternating between constructing and foraging. Some of the participants talked as they constructed, while others remained silent. However, all of us seemed to naturally drift into talking about the art once it became clear that construction had finished for everybody.

Luke's artwork (Figure 10.1) reflected the environment as he found it – organic and non-organic. Luke said that his art was an expression of his experience of the workshop. He stated that his circle of pine cones reflected the general theme of his current artworks.

Chloe (Figure 10.2) explored the theme of balance with a nest representing home positioned on a precarious see-saw. Home was a dominant theme for Chloe, expressing a great deal of interest in the houses and flats around the park and as to whether they were council or non-council. In addition, Chloe spoke about her desire to provide a 'home for insects'. The theme of harvest was also expressed through her use of colourful rosehips.

Generally, the group felt relaxed and at ease in their sharing. Photographs were taken of all the art work with the three participants sharing different feelings about leaving the art behind. Chloe expressed feeling vulnerable; worried her art would be kicked and stamped on. Luke was fascinated and amused by the thought of passers-by wondering about who had built the art objects and what they were about. This elicited a discussion about the relationship between artist and viewer in an art gallery context. Apart from the harvest theme, two other key themes did emerge. Firstly, the opportunity to try new things, secondly, participants registered their capacity to work far more spontaneously when using natural materials – standing in contrast to the greater planning undertaken back in the studio.

Winter

The members were introduced to the tradition that the winter solstice starts the twelve-day festival of Yule and related it to the moment when the wheel of the year is at its low point, ready to rise again. In Celtic tradition, the Yule celebration comes from the Celtic legend of the battle between the young Oak King and the Holly King. The Oak King, representing the light of the new year, tries each year to usurp the old Holly King, who is the symbol of darkness. We reflected on how these celebrations bring a momentary blaze of light into our lives, but also recognized that it can also be a difficult time of year as well. The art-making would be an opportunity to reflect or explore on their relationship with that time of year and perhaps share some common themes. Members were invited to create their own

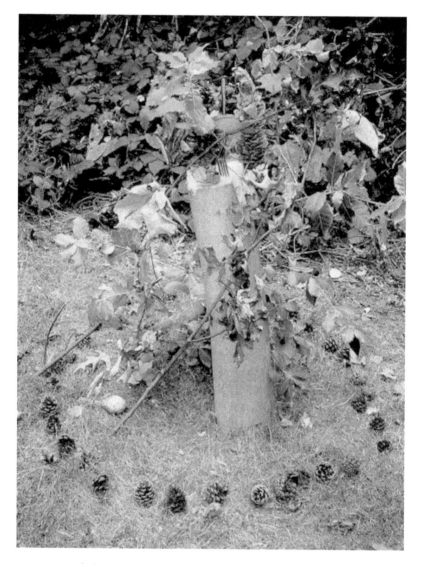

FIGURE 10.1 Luke's artwork

wheel of light. I provided a selection of candles for members to incorporate into their art-making. The first part was to be individual art-making; the second, an opportunity to make art as a group.

For the individual art-making, members left the circle to forage for natural art materials with the intention of bringing the materials back to construct their art work around the edge of the circle, creating the outside of their wheel. Members then had the opportunity to talk about their individual art and invite the thoughts

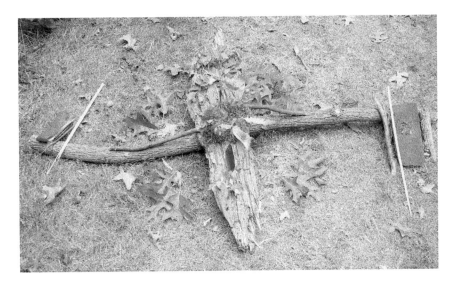

FIGURE 10.2   Chloe's artwork

and feelings of the other participants. After each person had received the feedback of others, they lit the candle(s) in their artwork. The candle symbolized the light they can receive from others and a reminder that they are not alone in the dark. For the group art-making, the members were invited to connect their individual art-making to the eternal wheel by constructing a piece together in the centre of the circle. After the artwork was completed the members lit the group candles together. As they lit the candles, the members were invited to share what they would wish to cast away into the darkness from this year and what hopes, dreams and wishes were waiting to grow in the coming year.

At the end of the workshop we explored how, despite the feasting, many of us experience winter as something to endure. We looked at how it may be useful to reframe winter as a period of waiting rather than a season where everything appears dead. The waiting process is an opportunity to connect with a feeling of stillness, a time to slow down rather than a time to fear that we will cease to exist. We considered that, even in the depths of winter, trees carry small buds that will eventually return as leaves. Waiting seems interminable and intolerable when we do not know if and when it will end. At this darkest point of the year we can be safe in the knowledge that we will see the light gradually return.

We explored that in the modern world there is an expectation that we must carry on in the same relentless pace no matter the time of year. By accepting our natural rhythms, like our need to sleep more and do less, we could perhaps alleviate the anxiety that there is something wrong with us at this time of year. We do not have to stop completely, just allow ourselves to slow down. With the returning sun, gradually we will be drawn out of our burrows and caves and into the light.

Spring

The theme of the spring workshop was the idea of emerging from the dark wait of winter into the light of springtime. Participants were encouraged to explore how the returning sun can generate new growth in their lives. Members were given some mythological background to Easter celebrations. They were offered the origins of the word Easter – the Anglo-Saxon deity Eostre, or Ostara, the goddess of fertility. Her feast, celebrated on the vernal equinox, is associated with the fertility symbols of eggs, rabbits and hares. (Cole, 2007, p. 42) The members participated in a visualisation meditation centred around imagining a seed uncurling in the warmth of the returning sun, fed by the surrounding natural springs (from which Springfield Park gets its name), releasing the tension of the long wait of winter.

Members were then invited to create their own celebration of the transformative power of spring. Together, the members built a large nest, big enough for them to stand within and where they would eventually place their individual eggs. Leading in to the making of their own eggs, the members were reminded that they stood at the spring or vernal equinox, the Celtic *Alban Eiler*, when the day and night are in perfect balance, and how from that day forward (until the autumnal equinox) the light will continue to grow. This was felt to be a time to awaken from hibernation, to start to move, grow and learn again; a time to celebrate personal growth in the past while looking forward to new growth in the future.

We deepened our exploration of the light and dark theme by considering the possibility of conflicting feelings, a tension between the need to burst out of one's current environment against the fear of embracing new experiences. We can feel a world full of light waiting to greet us, yet fear leaving one's safe place, the womb, the dark earth. There is no going back and yet there is the longing to return to the safety of the familiar. Members were invited to make an egg containing what is waiting to be born or even re-born within them. This provided an opportunity to explore what they felt was holding them back. Within the large nest the group then spent some time sharing their fears and desires.

In the final part of the workshops I invited them to draw upon the energy of spring to make the changes:

> *Like the seed pushing out of the ground,*
> *Blossom bursting from the carapace bud,*
> *The chick breaking from the shell,*
> *I invite you to break free of the containing egg, kick open the door, let the Sun in,*
> *Don't leave today by stepping out of the circle – break through it – kick or tear a*
>   *hole through the shell that surrounds you now.*

Some members readily kicked through the eggshell made of entwined sticks, whilst others were more hesitant pushing aside the sticks one-by-one. However, all of the members eventually stepped outside of their containing shell.

Summer

The summer solstice workshop invited studio members to celebrate their individual strengths using the traditional symbol of the oak. Studio members were also invited to explore the gifts they bring to collaborative activities using metaphors provided by honey bees.

After a grounding meditation, members explored the mythology and etymology informing the theme of the workshop. The oak was presented as having ancient connotations of strength and durability. To the Celtic people the oak held the true alignment of balance, purpose and strength. (Barret, 2010, p. 117) The oak is particularly prone to being struck by lightning. Most have the strength to continue to flourish after they have been struck. This gave them the association with the gods of thunder like Zeus and Thor. Members shared their associations with the durability of the oak, moments of great challenge when lightning had struck but they had survived. The group considered the strengths they could draw upon including their creativity. In mystic lore the acorn often represented the supreme form of fertility – creativity of the mind. This led to the first part of the art-making where members were invited to create a piece of art celebrating an aspect of their inner strength. A sharing of their creativity was then convened.

For the second part of the summer workshop, we turned to exploring the honey bee and the associated folklore throughout the ages. This included their role as messenger of the gods, that they were considered members of human families and emblems of sharing and cooperation (Barret, 2010, p. 130). Members were then invited to bring their individual strengths to the group by building a hive together imagining it as a receptacle for their collective strengths. The members used a variety of different materials found in the park to construct their hive.

Reflecting on all four Studio Upstairs workshops, members did make connections between the outside world and their inner world. Connections were also created between members through a shared experience of nature. In addition, the natural environment influenced the nature of the art that was made. The artwork was created more spontaneously, away from the aesthetic judgment of the studio, with greater expression of feeling. In my experience, this is a consistent theme when working with natural materials – they have a greater potential for client experimentation and play, leading to an enhanced experience of participation in group work. However, two potential members expressed a desire to participate but viewed the 'paganism' of the Celtic mythology as something with which they could not engage. Therefore, in designing subsequent workshops I endeavoured to keep the spirit of environmental arts therapy without including specific mythological narratives.

Mind in the City

In autumn 2015 and spring 2016 COATS was commissioned to run a series of art and nature well-being workshops by Mind in the City, Hackney and Waltham

Forest. We were approached by Mind to run these workshops due to the positive client feedback they had received from our Hackney pilot project in 2013. The workshops were to be part of the City and Hackney Wellbeing Network also using the Five Ways to Well-being model: "The network aims to help people to build resilience to prevent the onset of mental health problems and to alleviate issues such as stress, anxiety and low mood" (Mind in the City, Hackney and Waltham Forest, 2018). Participants were already registered with the network and invited to engage with the outdoor art-making according to their stated needs and interests.

In designing the well-being workshops, I endeavoured to incorporate Mind's understanding of their clients – centrally that they would probably be more comfortable using conventional art materials whilst engaging with nature. The clients that attended came from diverse backgrounds and were functioning reasonably well in their lives, but needed some support to prevent their mental health issues becoming more problematic. The participants all seemed to have had some previous connection or engagement with nature – either in this country or abroad. I was provided with trainee counsellors as co-facilitators for both the spring and autumn workshops. Whilst provision was made for eight participants, the average engagement for the autumn 2015 workshops was four people. For the spring 2016 workshop the participation rate was lower due to the unseasonably cold weather. The workshops lasted for two hours and were run over four consecutive weeks. They were created around four mental health areas that were central to the ethos of the Mind well-being network:

Autumn 2015

Managing Anxiety
Managing Depression
Improving Social Isolation
Managing Stress

Spring 2016

Managing Stress
Managing Anxiety
Managing Depression
Improving Motivation

I used natural themes and metaphors to help connect participants to each of the well-being areas. There was also a psycho-social element to each workshop, looking at common symptoms of each of the mental health issues. All the workshops include some form of art-making using conventional art materials. Each creative activity had to be easily replicable by the clients in their own time and have longevity over-and-above the immediate workshop rituals. I decided to use Springfield

Park again as my familiarity with its landscape would assist in facilitating a deeper connection for the participants and offer a more contained experience. (Part of this was due to the positive relationship I had developed with the park's ground staff.) All the workshops included an invitation to explore the park as a group, enabling the clients to create connections between the well-being theme offered and surrounding nature.

Autumn 2015 workshops

Autumn week one: managing anxiety

As the workshops coincided with the spring equinox, the twelve hours of light and twelve hours of dark provided a metaphor of mindfulness balance between positive and negative thoughts. Participants were invited to forage for two palm-sized objects representing light and dark. In the subsequent mindfulness meditation, participants were guided to think about a recent troubling event whilst holding an object in each hand: imbuing one object with an imagined negative outcome, the other object with a positive outcome. Participants were then encouraged to take a few moments to sit with the two possible outcomes held in both hands before physically dropping the negative object. To enhance the idea of letting go of thoughts, participants were asked to imagine the impossibility of an autumnal tree trying to hold onto its leaves. Participants then created leaves on which they wrote or drew negative thoughts they wished to let go.

Autumn week two: managing depression

Participants were offered the theme of connecting autumn's natural harvest with celebrating their own personal harvest. This was facilitated through art-making using conventional materials – the participants combining images of berries and fruits with elements of their life of which they felt proud. They also incorporated wishes for the new year or something that they wanted to bear fruit.

Autumn week three: improving social isolation

Through art-making and visualisations, participants were invited to explore the natural connections that surround them and their relationship to the wider natural world. Participants explored how feelings of isolation could be ameliorated through connecting with something larger than themselves. Within the meditation, participants were invited to visualise roots growing down to connect with the earth's very core, the source of the gravity that binds everyone to the planet, not just the centre of their world but everyone else's world.

For the art-making, the group was invited to create a natural entity or scene incorporating themselves into the picture and imagine the interconnections at work.

Autumn week four: managing stress

This included an invitation to create an ideal natural safe haven. This could be inspired by the guided visualisation that I provided, starting as a warm light in the centre of the body which then broadens out into a beautiful natural scene; perhaps something that the participants had seen in the park, an idealized natural location or a childhood memory. Participants were invited to return to this space in times of stress.

Spring 2016 workshops

Spring week one and two: managing stress and managing anxiety

These workshops followed the same rituals as those held in the autumn (see above for details).

Spring week three: depression

We discussed the value of regularly practicing gratitude to alleviate low mood using the energy of spring to kindle this habit. Spring offered an ideal opportunity for the participants to recount things in their lives that have blossomed into something good; a time when the seeds of their endeavours had come to flower or even a small thing that happened that day that had gladdened their hearts. Participants were invited to symbolise this by drawing plants and trees that blossom or flower – re-creating nature's celebration of life whilst thinking of aspects of their lives for which they would want to show gratitude.

Spring week four: improving motivation

Participants explored how low mood, stress or anxiety can diminish motivation to engage with everyday tasks. This included avoiding things that they feared and wanting to perpetuate feeling safe and comfortable. The egg provided an apt meta-phor for this situation. However, we also considered that the chick innately wants to break free of the safety of its shell. The guided meditation was built around this metaphor, incorporating the energy of spring to move towards greater fulfilment. Participants also drew pictures of eggs within nests and were invited to take the picture home. The image could then serve as a reminder to the participants to be kind to themselves, to nurture their ambitions both big and small.

Overall, the feedback from the participants was very positive. With the first round of workshops, the regular participants created connections with each other – offering peer support of shared experiences of mental health issues. The group spent time together after the workshops in the park café. Some expressed a greater motivation to regularly connect with green spaces. Some had not realised that Springfield Park existed and stated that they wished to return on their own time. Others requested ideas for additional outdoor well-being projects with which they could engage in the future.

Maryon Park community gardens

Summer 2016

Maryon Park Community Garden opened in 2012 and is a not-for-profit voluntary community project growing organic food in the Royal Borough of Greenwich. In April 2015 the Community Garden became a council-recognised constituted voluntary community group. Based in Maryon Park's former plant nursery, it provides raised growing plots to local people from diverse backgrounds who do not have gardens or for whom gardening can have health benefits.

The Community Garden now features fourteen growing beds, an orchard, a wild flower bank, art installations, a children's area, a poly tunnel, a greenhouse, cold frames, storage facilities and a garden meeting room that overlooks the park. The garden has an outdoor forest school classroom used by local primary schools and for COATS projects. The garden has regular open days and fund-raising events (which often include COATS children's outdoor art-making).

The garden feels like a hidden gem – a sanctuary within a sanctuary. The wider park has been nationally recognised through its Green Flag award. The garden is adjacent to the remnants of an Iron Age hill fort which was later exploited as a gravel pit. The park is a mixture of woodland, open spaces and activity areas.

The aim of the six summer workshops was to deepen participants' connection with nature through the senses:

1   Sight
2   Sound
3   Smell
4   Touch
5   Gravity (used instead of *taste* for health and safety reasons)
6   All the senses combined

I co-facilitated the workshops with my COATS colleague, Verity Blakeman. We decided that the workshops should offer a less directive approach than the previous two projects with a looser theme that allowed participants to connect with nature in a way that suited their own personal needs. Jordan offers an insightful perspective on working with the senses in nature:

> The therapeutic rational for participative experiences within nature is to encourage clients to awaken their senses. This is in order to address overall

patterns of relationality and to feel a connection with the more-than-human world. In doing this, part of the effect is to reawaken and understand human connections at the same time and how relationships take on different forms and have different feeling qualities.

(Jordan, 2015, p. 67)

The workshops' emphasis was on promoting well-being through facilitating the participants to explore and deepen their connection with nature. The workshops were advertised locally through posters and more widely using the online social networking site *Meetup*. Over the course of the summer it became apparent that a few of the participants had enduring mental health issues and experienced some isolation. One was recovering from a breakdown and another dealing with physical limitations.

The workshops started with a guided meditation to ground the participants in the space and to encourage them to focus on one of their senses to connect with their surroundings. This was followed by a mindful forage for natural art materials from the wider park. Participants were encouraged to use the featured sense, i.e. sight, hearing etc., to assist in their selection of art materials. We would then return to the garden to make art and share the experience. Whilst the art was posited as a way for the participants to express their connection with nature, unconscious metaphors relating to the participant's inner world consistently arose. As facilitators, it was our task to contain and regulate how deep the sharing went given the overall aim of the senses workshops i.e. promoting well-being rather than providing psychodynamic therapy. The participants exhibited a range of self-awareness and this was reflected in the depth of psychic material incorporated into the art. As Leah (pseudonym) stated:

> I found the COATS outdoor workshops very beneficial . . . The workshops helped me as foraging for objects to use in the art meant I looked around me and focused on what could be used, so absorbed my mind in that task. The walk around the park to collect them was calming too. Making art to convey feelings, thoughts and emotions was a good way for me to unlock things that were painful and hard to express in words.
>
> The 'sound' workshop was interesting as it was not just creating art (Figure 10.3) but had to be something I could play as well. I find music is very therapeutic as well. Anything that absorbed me fully in it, as I had to concentrate and tap into creativity, helped me while I was doing it to let my mind process and think about things that were uncomfortable in my life.

The Maryon Park workshops allowed the participants the space to instinctually connect with nature and their inner world. In contrast, the Studio Upstairs and Mind workshops involved a tightly structured format involving extensive preparation. With the Maryon Park workshops the work came through holding the space and being present to the needs of the participants.

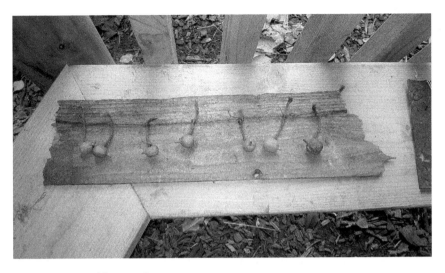

FIGURE 10.3 Leah's artwork

Conclusion

Through actively working in London's green spaces I am constantly reminded that the human relationship to the natural world varies greatly from person-to-person. However, connecting a diverse urban population to 'nature nearby' consistently involves the power of shared insight, ameliorating the loneliness of inner distress. Creating and facilitating a variety of appropriate workshops designed for an urban-based clientele, I have repeatedly witnessed the value of reconnecting with nature through the seasons and the senses. The core principles of environmental arts therapy can re-invigorate our sense of self and our connection to the natural world. In the British Isles, expressing the landscape of our inner world is often through a timely metaphor created from the seasonal weather. However, this is becoming more of a challenge as anthropogenic climate change disrupts the expected weather patterns, the extremes of which drive us away from positively engaging with nature.

All life springs from the Earth, not just our bodies but our minds and spirit too, finding natural expression in myth, metaphor and art-making. The value of the environmental arts therapy modality is the use of specific myth and ritual alongside the embodied engagement with Nature and the connections we can then make to our inner world. The very act of making art in green spaces, created from foraged natural materials that have existed for millennia, allows for unconscious elements to be made manifest. Emerging from the dark wood, we enter a clearing and a deeper understanding of ourselves and our place in the world comes to light.

Acknowledgements

Many thanks to my COATS colleagues, Tanya Andrew and Verity Blakeman for their support in writing this chapter and to the participants who contributed their experience.

References

Barret, L.G. (2010). *The tree mothers: Living wisdom of the ogham trees.* Marston Gate, Great Britain: Amazon Ltd.

COATS. (2018). Retrieved from: www.outdoorarttherapy.org.uk/.

Cole, J. (2007). *Ceremonies of the seasons.* London: Duncan Baird Publishers.

Cox, D.T.C., Fuller, R.A., Gaston, K.J., Hudson, H.L., and Shanahan, D.F. (2017). The rarity of direct experiences of nature in an urban population. *Landscape and Urban Planning*, 160, pp. 79–84. Elsevier. Open access article under the Creative Commons by license. Retrieved from: http://creativecommons.org/licenses/by/4.0/.

Government Office for Science. (2008). *Mental capital and wellbeing.* London. Retrieved 7 September 2018, from: https://assets.publishing.service.gov.uk/government/uploads/system/uploads/attachment_data/file/292453/mental-capital-wellbeing-summary.pdf.

Isserow, J. (2008). Looking together: Joint attention in art therapy. *International Journal of Art Therapy*, 13 (1), pp. 34–42.

Jordan, M. (2015). *Nature and Therapy.* Hove: Routledge

Mind. (2013). *Ecominds, feel better outside, feel better inside.* Stratford, London: Mind.

Mind in the City, Hackney and Waltham Forest. (2018). *City and Hackney Wellbeing Network.* Retrieved 7 September 2018, from: www.mindinhackney.org.uk/wellbeing-network.

Natural England. (2010). *Nature nearby*, p. 9. Natural England. Retrieved 7 September 2018, from: www.ukmaburbanforum.co.uk/documents/other/nature_nearby.pdf.

New Economics Foundation. (2008). *Five ways to wellbeing*, p. 12 [online]. Retrieved 7 September 2018, from: https://b.3cdn.net/nefoundation/8984c5089d5c2285ee_t4m6bhqq5.pdf

Studio Upstairs. (2017). Retrieved 24 September 2018, from: www.studioupstairs.org.uk/about/.

11

SPACE TO MOVE, EXPLORE AND CREATE

Taking art therapy into the outdoor environment in adult mental health services

Pamela Stanley

Introduction

Rust reminds us that indigenous people have always recognised that "we need a concept of self that describes how individuals are inextricably intertwined with community and earth" (Rust, 2009, p. 44). Living and working in Snowdonia I am very aware and connected to the natural cycles which affect and inspire my rhythms, creativity and sense of well-being. Being in nature helps me to 'feel' where and who I am and has led my interest in the therapeutic benefits of 'being' connected to the natural environment.

Environmental arts therapy practice moves from the boundaries of the art therapy room to work creatively in the natural environment. Here the main objectives are about being and experiencing, the development of restorative spaces and senses, as well as securing a safe environment, managing risk and supporting group dynamics. Jordan writes that to extend therapeutic practice outdoors we need to understand and "examine how the natural environment was separated from the psyche (and culture) in the first place" (Jordan, 2015, p. 18). Abram reminds us how sensuous engagement helps to "locate ourselves with the wider ecological matrix of which we are only part" (Abram in Jordan, 2015, p. 64). Like Schroeder, I became interested in understanding the deeper, hard-to-define experiences and values that people find in nature, which go by names like 'spiritual values' and 'sense of place' (Schroeder, 2008, p. 63).

This chapter provides an insight into the key stages and methodologies that have supported the development of an established environmental arts therapy practice within an Art Therapies Service in Adult Mental Health (AMH), Betsi Cadwaladr University Health Board, North Wales. By introducing the interrelationships between ecotherapy, ecopsychology and psychotherapy to explore how they have influenced and brought understanding to environmental arts therapy, this chapter offers insights, developmental approaches and fundamental knowledge. This has been inspired by a love of being outdoors and built upon many years' experience working with individuals and groups as an art psychotherapist in inpatient and community adult mental health services continually gaining an understanding of the Welsh language and culture. The development of environmental art therapy here in North Wales began by bringing nature into the art therapy studio before taking art therapy outdoors. The Art Therapy Outdoors pilot project (ATO.pp) was initially run for a period of six weeks with service users from the inpatient unit, within which I worked collaboratively with a like-minded occupational therapist experienced in outdoor education and research relating to both the call of the wild and risk management (Allfree, 2015). The positive outcomes of ATO.pp and the establishment of a regular Art Therapy Outdoors (ATO) service then went on to inspire the development of a six-month Community Environmental Arts Therapy pilot project (CEAT.pp). This was led in partnership with a Community Mental Health Team (CMHT) and their group coordinator, a mindfulness practitioner. A twelve-month Community Environmental Arts Therapy (CEAT) group was then also established based on the learning and success of the previous pilots with plans for continuation in the future.

My attendance of self-funded courses on ecotherapy with Haley Marshall and Martin Jordan in Derbyshire and on environmental arts therapy with Ian Siddons

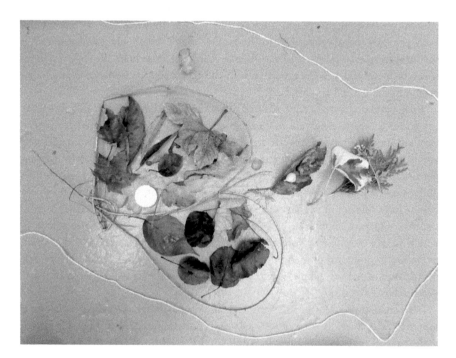

FIGURE 11.1   Heartfelt, a body map experience in response to December's descent in 2016.

Source: Art work by Pamela Stanley

Heginworth and Gary Nash at the London Art Therapy Centre, then gaining a certificate in Environmental Arts Therapy, supported this development. The ATO.pp and the CEAT.pp ran parallel to my training and were inspired by the book *Environmental Arts Therapy and the Tree of Life* (Siddons Heginworth, 2008). Sessions were based around the Celtic calendar and the Circle of Trees, following the yearly seasonal cycle and fostering a deep connection to nature, adapting themes as appropriate for each group. Creative activities, alongside ecotherapy ideas suggested by Sweeney (2013), were also a useful approach for awakening the heart and the senses and honouring both the masculine and the feminine principles. The aims were to reflect on experience, gain awareness and understanding of self and find a balance between doing and feeling within this pervasive Western culture. Sessions included creative art-making processes, ritual, storytelling and Welsh mythology and used the symbolism and metaphor which are abundant in the natural environment. This was described by a group member as "a space to move, explore and create".

> [S]o much that is true to ourselves must be felt first by the heart before it can be understood by the mind.
>
> *(Siddons Heginworth, 2008, p. 12)*

Environmental arts therapy framework

Siddons Heginworth states that *"environmental arts therapy is the therapeutic use of natural materials, natural locations, natural themes and natural cycles. At the heart of environmental arts therapy is the relationship between the natural world and the feeling self"* (Siddons Heginworth, 2008).

There are similarities between art therapy and applied ecopsychology which Sweeney suggests:

> are expressive modalities which seek the same outcome as conventional talk therapy ...", [but] "they attempt to address the gaps in more traditional verbal counselling through mediated exchange, via art or nature, of information between the repressed areas of one's personal psyche and one's conscious awareness.
>
> *(Sweeney, 2013, p. 13)*

> The body responds to an image of a thought or an idea first, before it responds to the words that describe that thought or idea.
>
> *(Sweeney, 2013, p. 14)*

Martin Jordan writes: "nature therapies have commonalities to the arts therapies which naturally work with the triangular relationship" (Jordan, 2015, p. 56). Jones describes how "nature is simply 'another room' or context for therapy" and "nature is 'co therapist' to the process, just as art-making is co therapist within traditional art therapy" (Jones, 2015, p. 11). The mental health charity Mind defines ecotherapy as including a wide range of practices which help improve mental and physical well-being by engaging in activities in nature. While other nature-based therapies may also include this, such as nature-guided therapies, horticultural therapy, Kaplan's restorative therapy (Kaplan, 1995) and adventure and wilderness, ecotherapy is a union between the ideas of ecopsychology and psychotherapy, exploring the relationship between ourselves, our connection to the natural world and the environment that we live within. It provides a solid theoretical, cultural and critical foundation for ecotherapeutic practice according to Buzzel and Chalquist (2009) who also cite Clinebell (1996) referring to healing and growing nurtured by a healthy interaction with the Earth. Jones states that:

> ecotherapists commonly hold two fundamental beliefs: (1) mental well-being is enhanced by being outdoors in the natural world (2) exploring the symbols, metaphors and narratives within landscape, the elements and Earth's natural resource is enriching spirituality and emotionally.
>
> *(Jones, 2012, p. 14)*

Casson writes that "metaphor 'carries across' an image, which may contain emotion, from the right brain hemisphere to the left brain, where the image is translated into language and thus conveys meaning" (Casson, 2004, p. 117). In this way metaphor acts as a bridge between 'inner and outer, self and other'. Casson further states that "metaphor occupies the transitional space spoken of by Winnicott as the place where creativity occurs." (Casson, 2004, p. 117).

Aims and theories informing outdoor practice

These included our standard art therapy aims:

1) to use creative art-making processes as a means of communication which do not depend on being verbally articulate or artistically correct
2) to use the space as a safe and confidential setting
3) to build up trust and to potentially share thoughts and feelings through creative expression which may be otherwise difficult to convey in words alone
4) to use the creative processes to express thoughts and feelings
5) to help individuals develop a sense of their own creativity
6) to enable a positive outlet for energy

(The Health Board's Bi-lingual Art Therapies Departmental Inpatient Art Therapy leaflet)

Yalom's (1995) 'eleven curative factors in group therapy' were also taken into consideration. There was also the opportunity for service users to experience what Potter and Connell (2005) describes as quiet time or 'mini solo'. Nicholls (2008) describes this as a form of privacy rather than isolation, a sense of solitude that was inclusive of experiences of "being alone together".

Art therapy is based on psychodynamic, attachment and group theories and this informed environmental art therapy service development to facilitate a safe, 'holding', Winnicott (1965) and 'contained space' Bion (1962). This is space where "a deeply felt wordless connection in nature or with a picture can facilitate the surfacing of a chain of subconscious emotions and memories. . . . and where thoughts and feelings can be explored and understood" (Sweeney, 2013, p. 13). Nature provides another tool for the art therapist's tool box, providing an array of materials and an added dimension to the therapeutic process, a natural creative space which is tangible and liberating. Importantly "nature provides a different form of emotional space" between therapist and service user "that can feel less threatening for service users who have poor relational experiences" (Jordan, 2015, p. 56). Of course, these environmental spaces can also be overwhelming, even threatening for some service users, and discussion on referral with the multi-disciplinary team is vital.

Through the development of a therapeutic relationship, the provision of a facilitating environment and engagement in the creative art-making process feelings may be expressed and reintegrated by projective identification. This is Winnicott's transitional space where the distinction between 'being' and 'doing' is experienced. Friedman (2004) presents a basic outline of Gendlin's approach to therapy based on 'focusing' or 'felt meaning'. Friedman cites Gendlin in saying "that the felt sense is crucial to psychotherapy" Friedman (2004, p. 24) and that

> psychotherapy begins when one makes direct reference to one's felt sense of the problem, issue, situation, or concern upon which one is working. By staying with the felt sense and finding a symbol that matches it, the felt sense unfolds its meanings and shifts. This felt shift. . . . is the feeling of therapeutic change actually happening.
>
> *Friedman (2004, p. 24)*

"Before we have explicit words, concepts, or other symbols, we understand the now viscerally through our experiencing of it". Experiencing is felt by the body, "rather than thought, known, or verbalized" Friedman (2004, p. 24). Bleakley suggests that "humans do not 'grow' unless they acknowledge their feeling states" Bleakley (1984, p. 73).

Initially, risk versus benefit needs to be assessed and therapeutic boundaries need to be clarified before each session to ensure safe practice, but once walking together outdoors the therapeutic relationship and process between therapist, service user and nature can feel much more balanced. Jordan describes being "together in a process of unfolding understanding which is creative and dynamic" and how 'moving along' together in a natural setting enabled unpredicted 'now moments' to occur, recognized as 'a moment of meeting' (Jordan, 2015, pp. 48–49). The frame is held by the quality of the therapeutic relationship relying upon the experience of the therapist and their internal sense of competence and self-confidence in holding the more dynamic and fluid process which unfolds in an outdoor context (Jordan, 2015, pp. 50–51).

In working with other agencies it was important to understand how to work collaboratively. Yalom (1995) raises the significance of needing to be familiar with the co-therapist, their different ways of working and behaviours and to ensure that there is time for reflection and discussion before and after group sessions. It is important for therapists to debrief and resolve any issues such as splitting and authority and for this to be noted and interpreted as necessary. Volunteer assistants received an induction, a role description and were involved in post group discussion and reflection. Working with a mindfulness practitioner raised questions as to whether it was more appropriate for thoughts to be expressed, accepted and let go of at each moment, or was it more beneficial to acknowledge and explore thoughts and feelings through the creative process to facilitate change.

The development of inpatient Art Therapy Outdoors in adult mental health services

Aims and format of Art Therapy Outdoors

The Art Therapy Outdoors pilot project (ATO.pp) for inpatient service users was based in and out of the art therapy studio for a six-week period, two hours a week. The aim was to combine walking, creativity and conversation in an alternative potentially restorative environment. The overall objective was to create a dynamic group process actively working with the mind and body, building personal awareness and strengthening individual functioning. Based on the findings of the pilot, the art psychotherapist and occupational therapist established the Art Therapy Outdoors (ATO) service using the same format and meeting regularly on a weekly basis. This offered some sense of constancy and continuity during what was otherwise a phase of insecurity and uncertainty for inpatient service users. Objectives were based on the experience of the established Community Outdoor Art Therapy Service (COATS) in London. These included offering a variety of media to be used to explore thoughts and feelings, some of which were familiar, others emerging through the creative process. The therapists provided a safe, non-judgemental natural environment for the group members to engage in. Many of the creative materials were found in nature, others were introduced because they complimented natural creativity such as clay, pastels, graphite, charcoal, paints and natural threads. Group members did not need to be 'good at art', but to get the most out of the sessions a willingness to engage with nature and experiment with creative materials was valuable. The therapists did not interpret the images, instead creating and sharing in the therapeutic group offered a space for reflection on the context of feelings. The therapists did however work with the group members to consider the impact of their past experiences on how they were feeling, responding and acting in the moment. The group itself also provided a safe therapeutic structure to gain better understanding of what was happening for the group members in the here and now.

Each session began with a brief introduction and the option to fill in an evaluation card. Some complimentary art materials, sketch books and a camera for communal use were carried each session; also, the first aid kit and mobile phones.

Practical issues were addressed such as the need to bring appropriate outdoor clothing and footwear. On arrival at the outdoor location some sessions began with a grounding exercise, based on mindfulness practice, to aid self-awareness and decrease anxiety. A flexible facilitated walk looking for and collecting natural materials for the creative processes followed; this encouraged physical exercise, social engagement, discovery and interaction with nature. Group members, either individually or together, engaged in the creative art-making process with natural materials either in the environment or on return to the art therapy studio. The therapists engaged with participants on a one-to-one basis and as a group when appropriate. Time was included for group reflection on their creative experiences and the issues that arose, both outdoors and on return to the studio. Group members were encouraged to fill in two authorisation forms, one for use of artwork/sound recordings and one for the Health Board's policy on photography and video consent. A copy of the images and words collected in the session was also printed and given to each participant as appropriate.

Referrals and risk assessment

Prior to each session a risk assessment for each location was completed. Referrals and risk were discussed with the multi-disciplinary team, ensuring individuals were physically able, had leave from the ward and no alternative commitments. An interest in the outdoors was preferable, with several group members having had some experience of art therapy. Themes were chosen to form a structure and aid boundaries. Weather and seasons influenced where each session was held, and phone signals were checked.

Locations and experiences

In North Wales there is an abundant and varied landscape close to the hospital, each space providing a unique experience of being in nature. The local university botanical gardens provided a less threatening, calmer environment with plenty of variety and interest. This offered a profusion of flora and fauna from all over the world; tropical, arid and temperate greenhouses; wild wooded areas and wild flowers; sweeping grassed lawns; a cascade and ponds; and a variety of plant beds. This was a feast for all the senses enabling the 'felt sense' to be discovered and experienced in a safe environment. Group members were able to move between wooded areas into wide open spaces, experiencing how movement and moods could change, voicing their relief or sense of freedom at emerging out into the open. There was opportunity for group cohesiveness, altruism and interpersonal learning. Giving and receiving were experienced in working creatively together sharing collective restorative moments when gathering autumn leaves or standing under the cherry trees, being showered by spring blossom petals. These were emotive, enjoyable and playful moments. There were calm times sitting on the grass listening to bird song under rustling bamboos, and reflective times when personal bundles were made and released down the cascade out to sea with collected tokens of hopes, wishes and letting go. The greenhouses were a welcome shelter when the wind blew and the rain fell, a warm retreat in winter weather, inspiring thoughts of journeys and cultures further afield. There was the continual metaphor of the seasonal cycles, and that change and renewal are always possible. The writing below was inspired by the vivid green heart-shaped leaves that grew when everything else all around was decaying underneath the trees. Words were gathered and collated together as we walked resulting in the narrative Heart Leaves describing the journey:

> *Peaceful, sunny, sparkle,*
> *Dazzling,*
> *Sadness, warmth.*
> *Heart leaves.*
>
> *Ravens, insects,*
> *Sun going, cooler,*
> *Quieter birdsong.*
> *Heartache.*
>
> *Raindrops glistening,*
> *River flowing,*
> *Tweeting birds.*
> *Heartfelt.*
>   *(Art Therapy*
>   *Outdoors session,*
>   *10 February 2016)*

We worked in other locations, including the shores of the Menai Straits, providing an ever-changing seascape. This is a nature reserve with paths through the trees and undergrowth, a fresh water pond and plenty of wildlife. A sheltered grassy glade and a blackthorn tunnel provided a white trail of blossom in spring leading out onto the shore and river estuary. The weather and the changing tides became a metaphor for feeling, giving a sense of freedom and wildness to the space. A disused slate quarry railway line provided a protected walk through mature woodland with carpets of flowers alongside a river, which led to up to local parkland overlooking the harbour.

Transportation and evaluation

Locations were approximately ten minutes' drive time from the hospital; the occupational therapy car was used to transport a maximum of three group members, due to capacity restrictions. The transitional driving period was positive, in that it gave service users an opportunity to talk and to prepare for being out in the community and then offered a quiet reflective time on the return journey. Evaluation and feedback were given verbally and there was continual liaison with the multi-disciplinary team both on the ward, at meetings and at the ward round. This was also written in service user integrated medical notes. On cessation of the ATO.pp a report was written, and service user reflection was collated using the postcards and recorded images (Stanley and Allfree 2014).

Co-facilitating and occupational therapy outdoors

As I was the sole art psychotherapist working in adult mental health services within the Health Board, the group was initially set up and co-facilitated with a colleague working in occupational therapy. It was important that we both understood our different approaches and individual ways of seeing. Profession and training, general interests and life experiences all added to what was brought to the group. Occupational therapists have embraced the identification and facilitation of meaningful engagement in activity to assist and manage illness and dysfunction. This includes skill acquisition, strength and endurance, cognitive strategies, social skills and empowerment, all considering the person, their environment, their performance and their spirituality. Holistic joint engagement with the service users in an outdoor natural environment through occupationally focused assessment enabled group members to identify opportunities for meaningful creative activity. Photographs were used as an aid memoir of previous sessions where continuation occurred. As time progressed ATO became an established collaborative service with occupational therapy, a working partnership, providing an opportunity for colleagues to learn and gain experience of environmental arts therapy.

Outcomes and group processes

Some of the group members developed in confidence and in their trust in being with others, which helped in gaining a greater understanding of relationships and behaviour. For some there was an improvement in communication skills and a greater understanding of self and those around them. The group enabled some members to find creative responses to difficult situations, improving self-esteem. It also provided opportunities for using and gaining awareness of all the senses, also a quiet natural space for reflection, or just 'being'. Members were able to enjoy the positive effects of engaging with nature in a meaningful way, building mindful personal awareness of the natural environment and restorative space. Members were able to express and share thoughts and feelings through the creative process and the use of metaphor, which may otherwise have been difficult to convey in words alone. The group provided a space for individuals to develop a sense of their own creativity and enabled a positive outlet for energy.

The development of community environmental arts therapy in adult mental health services

a) Community Environmental Arts Therapy pilot project

Based on the success of the inpatient art therapy outdoors service development, the community mental health team and the art therapies service identified a need for a time limited community environmental arts therapy group. The community mental health team group coordinator and the art psychotherapist invested in looking at ways to support service users, with emphasis on the continuity of care and alternative options to existing services. A six-month Community Environmental Arts Therapy pilot project (CEAT.pp) was set up and was proposed to run bi-weekly based in a central location. Extra time was scheduled for setting up the project and completing the final reports. The cost of facilitators and materials were paid from existing budgets, external room hire was paid for by extra funding through adult mental health services. The base room for the CEAT.pp was hired on the city outskirts which enabled service users to use public transport or their own vehicles, but this required therapists to transport some service users to the outdoor locations and tended to split the group and interrupt the therapeutic process during the travelling period. This interruption was offset by convening in the base room before and after each session for grounding and reflection. The group was facilitated by the art psychotherapist and the community group coordinator, a qualified and experienced mindfulness practitioner. Practicalities for therapists included mandatory training, car insurances, first aid, mobile signal, protective sun cream where appropriate, suitable outdoor clothing and umbrellas. The CEAT.pp included the participation of a volunteer artist with experience and an interest in art therapy, following the completion of disclosure and barring service (DBS) check, role description and induction. The same locations were used for the inpatient ATO group building on past experiences.

The aims of the community group were to:

1) provide access to art therapy in the community mental health services
2) give service users a chance to explore and understand difficulties with other people who have similar problems
3) help service users think about how powerful feelings affect behaviour, and how behaviour affects other people
4) provide a stepping stone towards engagement with friends and family and other important relationships
5) facilitate decision making, self-awareness and self-discovery enabling positive changes in life
6) help increase self-confidence and self-esteem

The CEAT.pp group members reported positive changes in themselves and in their relationships with others. They shared that the group could be beneficial and being outdoors could be enjoyable whatever the weather! Members felt optimistic about the therapeutic experience; they approved the facilitation of the group and there was acknowledgement of the value of being, changing, resolving and letting go. The majority chose to engage in mindfulness with some initially finding it difficult, but over time finding it beneficial. It was not always appropriate for some individuals, and creative alternatives and spaces were offered to group members on these occasions. Members participated in the creative art-making processes either using natural materials or complimentary art materials, working both indoors and outdoors. Confidence improved over time, as did the understanding of the use of symbolism, metaphor, ritual and stories to express thoughts and feelings. An example of how one member experienced the 'felt sense' was in his creation of a large circle of white daisies on the grass. This was made by picking all the ones from the inside and placing them on the outer circle, leaving a centre of green, with a small pile of leaves and twigs just inside the circumference. Through the embodiment of the creative process and gaining awareness of the symbolic meaning, he formed an understanding of needing to 'clear a space' in his life and begin to organise his current chaos. The pile represented the part that was difficult to get rid of, but he expressed feeling lighter at the end of the session (Stanley 2016).

b) The establishment of community environmental arts therapy

Following the evaluation of CEAT.pp, the collaborative art therapy and community mental health team partnership continued and an established twelve-month Community Environmental Art Therapy (CEAT) group commenced. This provided continuation of care, running as a bi-weekly slow open group, with the community mental health team group coordinator continuing as co-facilitator. Presentations based on the CEAT.pp report were given to other community locality meetings to raise awareness and resulted in referrals being received from various community mental health teams within the Health Board, with consideration that distances and geographical location could be a problem.

One of the discoveries from the CEAT.pp was that there was a need to find a base location in a natural setting for the group, hence relieving the necessity to move from the original base room to the outdoor locations. A stable base for the CEAT group was key to providing a safe shared space, offering continuity and constancy, and a local community run organic farm was sourced, which fitted the brief perfectly. There was a meeting room, an outdoor area with a fire pit and a hundred acres of land offering a varied environment of meadows, hills, streams, young and mature trees, orchards, bogs, protected wild areas, walls and hedges. Together with the allotments and animals there were safe footpaths suitable for all abilities. Public liability insurance and a risk assessment for the farm were already in place and an art therapy assessment was completed. Members were to make their own transport arrangements, which itself was part of the therapy process. A core group of members committed for the year attending bi-weekly with some new members being referred and others leaving at various times over the year. Overall, the group, the location and the format were successful even though there were some concerns over the future for the farm. Confidence grew as members became more familiar with the area and overall a cohesive group formed.

The CEAT group was also supported by a student nurse or the activities coordinator from the inpatient unit, to enable continuity during the occasional absence of one of the facilitators. Funding and support were received separately from the

Health Board's Arts in Health and Wellbeing service for an artist in residence, with an aim to exhibit and hang finished images on permanent display within the hospital. As a photographer, with a professional background in art therapy, the artist was able to use their mix of skills to sensitively capture the essence of the group in the natural environment over a few sessions throughout the year. This also provided a further dimension for reflection within the group as members were actively involved in the process of choosing the photographs produced.

Referrals and risk assessments

Referrals were received through the community mental health teams and therapy services. The criteria for referral identified individuals who had a history of complex, enduring, emotional and behavioural difficulties and who also had an interest in spending time outdoors in the natural environment. Some of the presenting problems of those who attended included: anxiety, assertiveness issues, post-traumatic stress disorder (PTSD), psychotic symptoms including schizophrenia, chronic depression, bi-polar disorder, personality disorder, self-harm and suicidal ideation, emotional bluntness, attachment issues, self-neglect and vulnerability. Assessment for suitability was conducted through a group assessment or individually with the referrer. Agreements and authorisation forms were signed during the introductory period.

Evaluation

An evaluation followed each session with reports provided for inclusion in community mental health team notes and feedback to care managers. Final environmental arts therapy reports were written on completion of both the CEAT.pp and the CEAT group. This included patient reflection, experiences and photographs. Individual final reports were sent to the relevant referrer, care coordinators, consultant psychiatrists and general practitioners. A personal discharge summary letter was sent to each group member. Information was collected over the period using Warwick Edinburgh Mental Wellbeing Scale (WEMWEBS) and/or CORE outcome measures and provided the team with a basic knowledge about service user's wellbeing and a continual risk assessment. The facilitators and volunteers had reflective time after each session where the group process was recorded and any concerns raised; further clinical and departmental supervision were attended as appropriate. Service users were contacted between sessions to maintain contact and provide encouragement as and when appropriate.

Outcomes, experiences and creative processes

Environmental arts therapy artwork included the creation of castles made of twigs and propped against trees, some with flowers scattered over the top. Group members bravely felt and faced their fears through the creative process enabling the expression and sharing of painful experiences. There were other castles with hidden doorways camouflaged in the bracken, gently inviting. Another open 'mapped out' castle was spread over a soft mossy rock, another had petals decorating a large tree trunk and encasing a symbolic welcoming feast of berries on bark plates. This was a 'home', a 'safe space', a symbolic representation of personal boundaries. The "shadow self" was explored based on Jung's ideas that everything in nature has an equal and opposite side; his concept of a shadow that represents the subconscious part of the psyche. Sweeney writes that while the "shadow self" contains the darker, shameful and frightening feelings about ourselves, the "golden shadow" contains the fear of being too good, too powerful or too spectacular which is often submerged and denied (Sweeney, 2013, p. 90). Photography was a preferred creative process for one group member who captured the shadow image of the whole group giving them and himself a feeling of inclusion and self-worth. Sound drawings (sounds represented in various shapes and colours) helped members connect to their sense of hearing. There was increased awareness of all the senses, smelling herbs, seeing colours and shapes in the flowerbeds, hearing the birds, feeling the hardness of rocks and the softness of the clay. The trees were always engaging, tasting red rosy apples, sensing the enormity and strength of the ancient oak trees and the promise in their acorns, the young slender ash groves, the touch of the papery silver birch bark, and the ever-present rosebay willow herb changing in splendour throughout the year sharing with us all its appearances and characteristics on our journey. There were smells of earthy fungi, the softness of ferns, deep pools and flowing streams, rows of fruits and vegetables, seeds, wild berries and blossoms.

There were times to acknowledge transition, moving from the feeling of being stuck in a damp bog to free-flowing waters, recognising the continual flow and changes of the rain cycle and of life. Mobiles were made relating to personal balance, heavy stones weighed against numerous twigs and sticks, sparse leaves and ferns fragile against strong tree trunks, swaying in the breeze, suspended from boughs or tucked into forked branches. There were expressions of frustration, sometimes a sense of achievement, feeling and seeing how balance can shift where it needs to move and how this related to other aspects in life. There was the crossing of thresholds through trees and branches and the building of bridges, with both the physical and metaphorical crossing from one side to the other. Labyrinths were spread out over the meadows or gently created under a tree, each a meaningful experience shared with feeling. There was the opportunity to make physically difficult outward journeys and return needing inner strength and outer support. There were times around the fire pit creating crowns for kings and queens, finding a voice through ritual and enjoying creative play.

Group members described their experiences of environmental arts therapy using words such as compassion, empathy, kindness, joy, playfulness, friendship, altruism, learning, hearing, speaking, doing, being, explorative, reflective, space and containment. They described meeting their challenges with words such as tears, sadness, overwhelmed, anger, fear, adventurous, courageous, stoic and resilient. They used phrases such as "rediscovery of creativity", "the influence of others", "giving and receiving", "air, fire, water, earth" and "warrior spirit". Feedback included their experiences of working collaboratively and the joint creation of a mandala using gathered natural materials encouraged a sense of belonging and the feeling of being a part of something special (Stanley 2018).

Conclusion

This chapter described the development of environmental arts therapy practice in adult mental health services which successfully moved from the boundaries of the art therapy room to explore creatively in the natural world outdoors. Being in nature provided distinct therapeutic benefits where meaningful personal experience, the development of restorative inner and outer spaces and the awakening senses can be managed within a safe shared environment. By understanding and drawing upon the different perspectives of co-facilitators alongside continual risk assessment made it possible to create boundaries outside in nature and manage diverse group dynamics.

A space was provided that allowed for connection or reconnection with the natural environment and the annual cycle and it became apparent how this affected mood and senses, the active masculine and the feeling feminine. Being outdoors in natural surroundings offered an opportunity to engage with the 'felt sense', enabling heart felt moments to occur, with the consequent gaining of self-awareness and the facilitation of change. New insights emerged as walking side by side outdoors changed the dynamics and status of the therapeutic relationship. Natural metaphors all around facilitated awareness and understanding, visually and verbally, with an array of natural materials allowing creative processes to be discovered, explored and experienced. Group interaction enabled personal understanding, the joy of giving and receiving, playful experiences and learning with others. Yet there was also time within the group setting for individual reflection.

New insights were given to practitioners around working spaces, individual service users and the joys and challenges of being outdoors learning new ways to create boundaries in the outdoor environment and further understanding of safety and risk factors. Liaising with the service users and referrers to ensure being well informed prior to sessions, alongside continual physical and mental assessment, proved vital. Understanding the different opportunities provided by locations and the discovery and use of 'wilder' spaces came with experience and self-confidence. Being outdoors sometimes made 'containing' and 'holding' the group more challenging, but it provided increased opportunity for service users to engage and connect with nature and allow 'now moments' and 'moments of meeting' to occur facilitating self-discovery Jordan (2015). Chief among outcomes were a sense of hope and optimism. Group members did not feel alone with their problems, instead learning with and through others was achievable and helping each other gave a sense of value and worth. Members were able to discover and reflect on family issues and childhood events within the safety of the group. There was the development of social skills including tolerance and empathy and working together enabled cohesiveness and a sense of belonging and acceptance. The use of creative processes facilitated the releasing of suppressed emotions and disclosure within the group with the consequent growth of understanding, learning how to live as part of something larger than oneself.

The use of pilot projects offered vital knowledge and confidence for this innovative practice and assisted greatly in the development of both the inpatient and the community environmental arts therapy groups resulting in an established service. In addition, the support of appropriate clinical supervisors, arts therapies departmental support, time for reflection after sessions with co facilitators and managerial backing was essential.

The nomination for the Health Board's 'new ways of working' award helped to raise the profile and gain further support. To make possible further development across the Health Board it is now recognised that managers and therapists need to work together and resources need to be made available for training opportunities and clinical supervision to continue safe and innovative practice. The service manager of Adult Mental Health services supported the community development by stating "... *not only does it provide a stepping stone from inpatient based care to the home, but it allows individuals to explore and connect with their own neighborhoods in a meaningful way*". The head of operations and service delivery added that

> Not everybody can use words to articulate who they are and how they experience the world and we have an accountability to move beyond traditional methods of 'talking' if we want to make services as accessible and person centred as possible . . . patients and therapists need safe, secure, consistent places to work in.

Nature proved to be just this, a safe, secure and consistent place for us to work in, 'space to move, explore and create', but it was so much more than this as well. Jung describes this perfectly when he writes that

> At times I feel as if I am spread out over the landscape and inside things, and am myself living in every tree, in the splashing of the waves, in the clouds and the animals that come and go, in the procession of the seasons.
>
> *(Jung, 2008, p. 35)*

References

Allfree, S. (2015). *Call of the wild: Is it always about risk? A meta-ethnographic approach.* MSc Dissertation in Occupational Therapy, Bangor University (Unpublished).

Bion, W. (1962). *Learning from experience.* London: Karnac Books.

Bleakley, A. (1984). *Fruits of the moon tree: The medicine wheel and transpersonal psychology.* Bath: Gateway Books.

Buzzell, L., and Chalquist, C. (2009). Introduction: Psyche and nature in a circle of healing. In *Eco therapy: Healing with nature in mind.* Berkeley, CA: Counterpoint.

Casson, J. (2004). *Drama, psychotherapy and psychosis: Drama therapy and psychodrama with people who hear voices.* Hove, East Sussex: Brunner-Routledge.

Clinebell, H. (1996). *Healing ourselves, Healing the Earth.* New York: Haworth Press.

Community Outdoor Art Therapy Service (COATS). Retrieved from: www.outdoorart therapy.org.uk.

Friedman, N. (2004). Retrieved from: www.americanpsychotherapy.com.

Jones, V. (2012). Practice definition: Art therapy outdoors. *Newsbriefing,* June, pp. 14–15.

Jones, V. (2015). The greening of psychotherapy. *Newsbriefing,* July, pp. 10–13.

Jordan, M. (2015). *Nature and therapy: Understanding counselling and psychotherapy in outdoor spaces.* London and New York: Routledge.

Jung, C.G. (2008). *The earth has a soul: C. G. Jung on nature, technology and modern life.* Berkeley, CA: North Atlantic Books.

Kaplan, S. (1995). The restorative benefits of nature: Toward an *integrative* framework. *Journal of Environmental Psychology,* 15, pp. 169–182.

Mind. Retrieved from: www.mind.org.uk.

Nicholls, V. (2008). Busy doing nothing: Researching the phenomenon of "quiet time" in a challenged-based therapy program. *Journal of Experiential Education,* 26 (1), pp. 8–24.

Potter, T., and Connell, T.O. (2005). The use of solo in Canadian college and university outdoor education and recreation programs. In Knapp, C.E., and Smith, T.E. (Eds.), *Exploring the power of solo, silence and solitude* (pp. 137–150). Boulder, CO: Association of Experiential Education.

Rust, M-J. (2009). Why and how do therapists become eco therapists? In Buzzell, L., and Chalquist, C. (Eds.), *Eco therapy: Healing with nature in mind* (pp. 37–45). Berkeley, CA: Counterpoint.

Schroeder, H.W. (2008). The felt sense of natural environments. *The Folio,* pp. 63–72.

Siddons Heginworth, I. (2008). *Environmental arts therapy and the tree of life.* Exeter: Spirit's Rest Books. www.environmentalartstherapy.co.uk.

Stanley, P. (2016). *Community environmental art therapy pilot project report.* Betsi Cadwaladr: University Health Board, Art Therapies in Adult Mental Health.

Stanley, P. (2018). *Environmental art therapy community group report.* Betsi Cadwaladr: University Health Board, Art Therapies in Adult Mental Health.

Stanley, P., and Allfree, S. (2014). *Creative art therapy group outdoors pilot project report.* Betsi Cadwaladr: University Health Board, Art Therapies in Adult Mental Health.

Sweeney, T. (2013). *Eco-art therapy: Creative activities that let the Earth teach.* ISBN 0-6159-0147-6.

Winnicott, W.D. (1965). *The maturational processes and the facilitating environment.* London: Hogarth Press Ltd.

Yalom, I. (1995). *The theory and practice of group psychotherapy* (4th edition). New York: Basic Books.

PART V

Elders and endings

The wild road on

12

TREES OF LIFE AND DEATH

A journey into the heart of Transylvania
to use environmental arts therapy with
groups of adults and staff in palliative care

Hannah Monteiro

Introduction

Before sharing my reflections on the environmental arts therapy workshops delivered, it seems appropriate to give context to the country, season, culture and hospice. It had long been in my heart to return to Romania, as I had lived there for a semester as an Erasmus student and had grown fond of the location and its people. I wished to revisit the medieval city of Braşov in the Transylvanian region. It is a place surrounded by citadel wall ruins, bear filled mountains and howling wolves in dense green forests. My arrival was greeted by an immense downpour of rain that was followed by hot and balmy end of July days, but autumn seemed to be peeping through the cracks during the month of August. The leaves were already changing colour and beginning to fall, yet still enough heat remained for summer to hold on. In the depths of this beautiful place, I was aware of the numerous people harmoniously working and knowing the urban and rural landscape. It was common to see a horse and cart passing by carrying the harvest and from a distance the faint movement of a shepherd and his sheep on the hillside.

Transylvania and Romania, as a whole, are embedded in spiritual traditions and folklore. Romanians predominantly follow the Orthodox Christian Church where great importance is placed on ceremonies to mark the rites of passage including birth and death. There is a belief amongst many that baptism in water purifies the soul from sin, renouncing the devil (Fosztó, 2009). I was informed by a local that in Romanian folklore a person who dies unbaptised is vulnerable to become corrupt and turn into a vampire. This myth undoubtedly inspired the famous gothic horror novel *Dracula* written by Bram Stoker in 1897. The story tells of how human blood becomes the vampire's elixir of life and it exposes the human fear of death and the unknown and the fantasy of immortality. Another well-known Romanian fairy tale that is routed in those themes is *Youth without Age and Life without Death* written by Petre Ispirescu in 1862 (cited Teodorescu, 2015). The story depicts a young prince, an only child, who leaves the palace and his parents to journey to a foreign land outside of time that gives the gift of youth and self-continuation. It unfolds that one day during his stay in this magical land he enters the forbidden valley, "The Vale of Tears". Instantly his heart aches with a yearning to be reunited with his parents. The prince travels back to his homeland where time does not stand still, and his parents have long since been dead. He too then meets death. The fear of death and the desire to sustain life are strong motifs expressed in numerous fairy tales, stories and myths of this culture. These themes naturally emerged in my work at the hospice, together with the avoidance of allowing death as a subject of conversation.

Transylvania's scenic landscape and captivating culture remains a tourist attraction. However, it is also a place where the cobwebs of communism linger and evidence of its history and struggles can still be seen and felt in the retelling of people's personal stories. After the fall of communism in the country the first palliative care service, Hospice Casa Speranței (Home of Hope) was created; prior to this no provisions were given to the terminally ill (Mosoiu Andrews Perolls, 2000). The hospice provides holistic palliative care for both adults and children with incurable illnesses and support for their families. It was in the grounds of this hospice that I delivered environmental arts therapy workshops for groups of outpatient adults attending the day-care centre as well as to hospice staff from the multi-disciplinary team.

The day-care provision offers a space to rest, relax and socialise, whether conversing over a meal with each other and staff, enjoying an arts and craft activity or participating in a relaxation workshop. Five different groups of adults attended weekly, one group for each day of the week and there were eight to twelve patients per group. My work with the patients took place over a three-week time frame. During the first week I attended each day-care group to give me the opportunity to introduce myself and the workshops, build rapport and observe the group dynamics. In the second week, I facilitated the patients to create their 'Tree of Life'. The final week was set aside for the patient groups to reflect on the metaphorical storms that affected their trees and how they might overcome them. I was supported by health and social care staff who, being fluent in English, also acted as translators due to my limited Romanian.

In the final week, staff were offered two self-care environmental art therapy workshops between one to two hours long depending on the needs and size of the staff group and the consequent time constraints. Each workshop contained six to ten participants drawn from a variety of different disciplines: administrative, medical, social work and managerial. Environmental arts therapy offers natural materials (used indoors or outdoors), natural themes and natural cycles as a sensory canvas upon which the client can express themselves creatively, in context with the turning year.

The Tree of Life

The 'Tree of Life' model (Ncube Denborough, 2008) is a narrative psychosocial approach enabling a reflective and healing process whilst minimising the risk of re-traumatisation. I decided to adopt this model for the patient workshop, as it has been successfully conducted around the world with adults and children who have experienced various life traumas. Furthermore, due to its visual and metaphorical nature it has the ability to bridge language barriers.

The Tree of Life is a two-part model that I split into two separate workshops for each patient group. Firstly, participants are invited to create the image of a tree as a symbol of themselves enabling them to reflect on their situations, strengths and difficulties. The second part of the model invites the participants to put their trees together to form a forest and to share what 'storms their trees have endured' (what life stresses and traumas have affected them) and how their tree 'weathered the storm' (how they coped with these difficulties).

For the first set of workshops, as a reference point to aid the participants I created a visual template of a tree with the different points for reflection labeled in Romanian.

Rădăcini, Roots: family history and heritage, culture and country

Solul, Soil: where you live, daily activities, hobbies

Trunchi, Trunk: your strengths, personal resources, adaptability

Rămuri, Branches: hopes, dreams, wishes, objectives

Frunze, Leaves: the people who are important to you, your family, friends or others that you care about. These may be people in the present or in your past.

Fructe, Fruits: the gifts that you have received from others or that which you would like to give to others. These things might not necessarily be material, but may include love, kindness and time spent with people.

Following the explanation of the visual template, I invited participants to explore the array of art materials and foraged natural woodland materials to find items that they would like to become part of their Tree of Life. The woodland feast was a mixture of summer's last green vegetation and flowers and autumn's first fruits and colour-changing leaves. Participants were then given space to start making their tree before I offered any supportive input.

During the making of the trees, several conversations were naturally happening between participants around the table at the same time. Despite having interpreters, to some extent communication was still problematic. Although all conversations directed between myself and the participants were translated, I had not considered the fact that working in groups meant that several conversations were happening simultaneously. It was therefore impossible for all of this to be translated back to me and I noticed how I was trying to compensate by looking at facial expressions and body language for what my ears could not understand.

I interpreted a variety of responses to these first sets of workshops. Some patients seemed intrigued or excited by the making of their tree whilst others appeared more tentative and needed encouragement from staff to initiate participation. Additionally, some patients wanted to sit at the table and watch others work but not take part, and others chose not to take part and sat away from the making table. Through a combination of encouraging group discussions, individual conversations (via the interpreter) and anonymous written feedback, I was able to gain more insight into how the participants were finding the workshops.

Collectively the group shared that creating their Tree of Life felt relaxing, nostalgic and an enjoyable experience to share alongside others. Even though every conversation around the table was not translated, I witnessed the interactions that participants had with each other and there appeared to be poignancy and power in the making and sharing of the story of their Tree of Life. Their trees provided a relatable metaphor from which conversations seemed to grow, concerning who they were and about their life stories.

As the translator and I went around the participants individually, some shared about their evolving Tree of Life and how different materials symbolically represented aspects of their personal life. Being able to speak via the translator to individual participants, I felt able to support them with their process and thinking. Written feedback forms offered another and perhaps safer way for participants to share both their positive and negative experience of their workshops. One participant wrote, "the Tree of Life is associated with my family but given our situation it doesn't make sense anymore." Another participant shared, "While I was drawing the tree, I felt great and I remembered my childhood. At the beginning I was resistant to making anything as I didn't know how to start, then I allowed my imagination to lead and did what I was imagining."

The leaf of death

In one patient group, whilst making their trees, a particular leaf was being passed around the table and its beauty was admired. The leaf had begun its autumnal change and its greenness had started to transform into a bright golden yellow with a hint of glowing orange. This leaf sparked a conversation about what autumn meant to people. Some spoke about the beauty in the myriad of colours and the fruitful harvests. Others spoke about autumn being a warning that the bitterly cold Romanian winter was coming, and all things were starting to die. This was the first time that the group was able to talk together about death, albeit the death of nature, not their own. Sharing their feelings about the turning of the seasons became an outlet for reflecting together on mortality and the transience of life. The group asked that I try to preserve this leaf in its beautiful colour and shape. A participant passed me the glue and I began the meticulous process of coating the leaf. This preservation process felt reminiscent of the fantasy themes of perpetual youth and immortality in *Dracula* and in *Youth without Age and Life without Death*.

During the second set of workshops, the group who had discovered the beautiful leaf requested to see what had happened to it one week later. The entire leaf had died and although it had stiffened with the added strength of the glue, its shape and beautiful colours had been lost and it had curled up. The group appeared saddened by this and the once admired leaf was no longer passed around. I was left holding what I felt to be the 'Leaf of Death', the very thing that the patients did not wish to talk about, whilst the group admired their 'Trees of Life'. The juxtaposition of the dead leaf and the vibrant living tree compositions left me feeling silenced.

In my silence (noted in my diary) I spoke to the leaf:

> *Leaf*
> *of death*
> *I watched you*
> *as your colours changed*
> *and I marvelled at your beauty*
> *but no matter how much*
> *I coat you in preservative*
> *I cannot keep you*
> *as you are*

I felt like a failure to the patients and to the leaf, as I had been given the job of preserving life and I had not succeeded in saving it.

In the second set of workshops each group was invited to place their trees together to talk about the metaphorical 'storms' that affected their lives and how they overcame them. No group wished to talk about their storms as a cohort. Most expressed fear about what might come out if the group talked about their difficulties. They discussed how they only wanted to reflect on the good things in their lives. However, some participants spoke to me about the challenges that they faced as I went around the table speaking to individuals with my translator. One individual annotated their tree with a poem (see Figure 12.1) which translates as:

> *A weary tree*
> *Is laying at my feet*
> *Defeated by the ending night's storm*
> *Then the travelling clouds run fragile*
> *Sunlight timidly clothes the forest*

This poem was read out to me in Romanian and although I had to wait for its translation, I could see from the facial expression of the poet that creating this tree and the accompanying words enabled her to find some meaningful expression about her life journey. It seemed to me that this participant clearly related to the personification of a tree, and through this was able to reflect on her relationship to her terminal illness and life challenges. That is, as a 'weary tree' she lay down feeling 'defeated' by the 'storm'. Nonetheless she drew some comfort from the 'fragile clouds' and the 'timid sunshine' (perhaps a hint of the hope that lies in the continuation of things) and from being a part of the forest, she shared feeling a sense of belonging, unified with the other patients.

The placing of the trees together in 'a forest' was a group process and seemed to evoke a lot of emotion (see Figure 12.2).

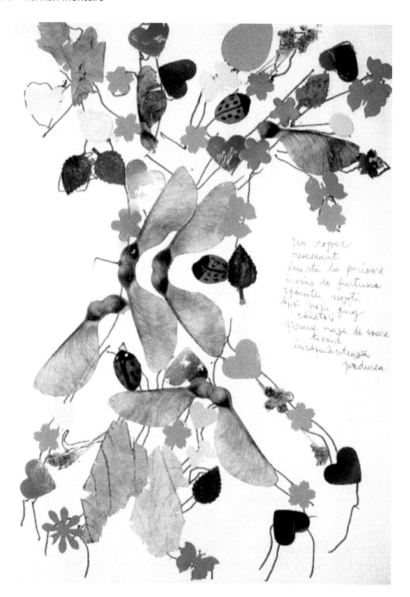

FIGURE 12.1 A weary tree

Whilst the project began as an individual reflection, there was often a clear trans-formation when one tree on its own became a part of this forest. Many participants spoke about the beauty in the trees being together in this way, yet each tree still being an individual. One participant shared:

It was an enjoyable experience to make my tree, but to see the trees all together in their forest was a proud moment, where I felt as though I had a place where I belonged.

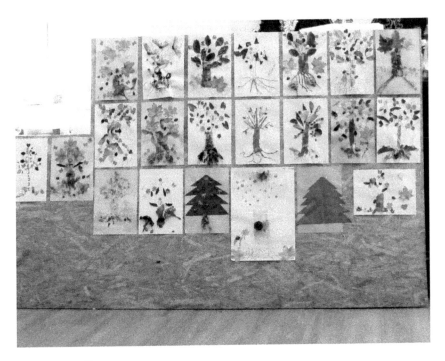

FIGURE 12.2 Forest

This patient spent a long time standing in front of the forest smiling with tears in her eyes as she shared how this 'togetherness' had made her feel. She expressed that having a terminal illness can make one feel alone, but (like the poet above) seeing her tree amongst the other trees meant she no longer felt alone.

Staff environmental arts therapy workshop

As I approached the end of my time at the hospice, I facilitated two environmental arts therapy workshops for staff groups using natural foraged materials and clay donated by a local potter. One workshop was conducted outside in the hospice garden and the other inside the day-care centre due to the weather conditions. I invited the staff to create something of their choice, to creatively express their thoughts and feelings on what it is like for them to work in the hospice. Following the making of their creations there was an opportunity to share these reflections as a group. I too decided to join in the making and reflecting process.

The inspiration for these staff workshops evolved as a result of a conversation with a member of staff who shared that she loved her job but felt on the brink of burn-out. She expressed how distressing it was to repeatedly witness the difficult circumstances patients faced and the death of many people she cared for. Personally, I noticed how staff came in every day smiling. Although I could see that there was a love and passion in their patient care, I wondered what other feelings might be behind their smiles. Val Huet (2017) stresses the dichotomy between staff maintaining a composed demeanour and the suppression of their true emotional reality, thus making their hidden feelings difficult to address. Likewise, and perhaps in response, the patients seemed to parallel this process, sometimes hiding their own distressed thoughts and feelings and upholding the appearance that all is well. To some extent I hoped that the environmental art therapy workshops could offer space and some containment for these more challenging feelings.

Naturally, working with the staff group had a very different feel to working with terminally ill patients. Additionally, the majority of staff could speak English and did so for my benefit. It made such a difference to be able to understand what was being spoken around me. Whether or not the conversation was directed at me, speaking the same language helped me feel more connected to the staff group and the creative process.

Whilst making art, the conversations around the table were focused around their feelings about work and how their day had been, as well as sharing about themselves and their families. All the staff admired the banquet of materials, helping themselves according to their appetite for colour, texture and shape. There seemed to be excitement, curiosity mixed with a little anxiety about what the workshop was and what feelings it might bring.

Even though there was no obligation to make or to share, both tasks brought up ambivalent feelings for the staff. All shared how thankful they were to be given an opportunity to be creative together. A new member of staff further expressed how the workshop had helped her to get to know her colleagues better. Even so, one participant shared that whilst they had really enjoyed the time spent creating artwork amongst colleagues, they did not feel comfortable sharing their personal thoughts and feelings with the others. It appeared that self-reflection and sharing was not always part of the staff's established role in the hospice, and the experience was strange, uncomfortable and exposing for some.

Staff agreed that they consistently put the needs of their patients first and reflected on how they often left their own needs and overwhelming feelings of loss behind. The desire to not have to carry some of the emotional burdens home was shared by some. They described how engaging in the workshop felt as though they had managed to break away from their routine and 'steal' some time for themselves. It was reflected that this workshop was "a time, like in childhood, where we were the centre of the action". Some participants expressed that they had not made anything since kindergarten and relished the opportunity. There was a lovely sense of mischief, laughter, mess and play, as if the natural materials were a midnight feast at a young person's sleepover! Perhaps rekindling childhood insecurities, some staff expressed feelings of frustration at what they considered to be their lack of ability to create aesthetically pleasing artwork. Others felt stuck for some time, not knowing what to make. The staff worked through these barriers in different ways. Some appeared to take inspiration from their colleague's creations, while others used their phones to research for ideas on the internet, feeling safer in copying a found image. The remaining staff contemplated quietly, found inner inspiration and then began to create.

The clay was very popular; this was summed up by a member of staff who said, "I enjoyed the activity, especially working with clay, which was new to me and I had always wanted to do it". Another participant shared that the process of kneading and molding the clay felt therapeutic and relaxing, as if through the clay they were giving themselves a hand massage. It was agreed that working with clay brought about a sense of feeling cathartic at the end of their day and something they would particularly like to do again to assist with self-care. Whilst there was a variety of artwork created, many had made containers and nests out of the clay and natural foraged materials. Some creations were wide and open, so that it was possible to see clearly inside, others were semi-open and contained partially hidden woodland treasures (see Figure 12.3). One was made like a closed envelope with its content hidden. In the sharing time we reflected together on this container theme and saw how containers were an appropriate metaphor for people who had to hold so much. Staff felt that the process of building nests was expressing a part of them that wished to protect and nurture the people in their care. They expressed how this workshop had helped them identify and understand this shared need.

The return of the leaf of death, now honoured in beauty

I brought the 'Leaf of Death' (given to me by one of the adult groups) to work on in the staff making and reflecting sessions. This leaf continued to carry my frustration and anger at not being able to halt the dying process. The attempted preservation continued as I covered parts of the leaf in salt, but all the salt did was cling to its shell and expose the waterless veins in its body. I recognised in myself a process in which anger at my inability to preserve the leaf eventually moved into acceptance. This leaf originally had been brightly coloured, supple, flat and alive, but in its dying the colour faded, it dried out and it curled up. Where at the beginning I had worked to preserve the leaf, now my approach changed, and I started working with its shape in death. In its sadness and beauty, the curled leaf became a metaphorical container for my own feelings on life, dying and death. Its outside represented my original feelings of frustration and anger captured in the coating of glue and salt. Its inside held my tears of sadness that the ill and dying patients could not see – tears that metaphorically fell into the leaf like cascading droplets of pearls and glistening gold. Finally, I placed an opening horse chestnut seed beside the closing 'Leaf of Death' the beginning and the ending of life seemed harmonious together (see Figure 12.4).

The leaf expressed my acceptance of death and the privilege that I felt in working with this client group – the return of the 'Leaf of Death' was now honoured in beauty. The composition as a whole for me held all that is precious about working in palliative care – the beauty, the fragility, the sadness and the sacred.

My time at Hospice Casa Speranţei was humbling and enriching; I met a staff and patient community who were resilient and had formed strong supportive relationships. Yet, amidst this, I also experienced an environment where death was ever present but barely talked about. However, just like in the weaving together of life

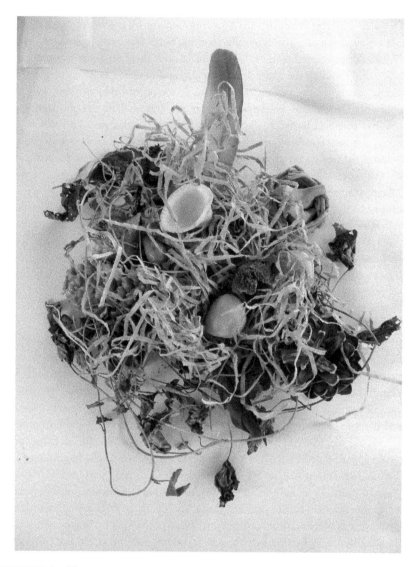

FIGURE 12.3 Nurture

and death in fairytales, the environmental arts therapy workshops had given both patients and staff a medium and a language in which they could express and share feelings of grief, loss and hope.

The workshops themselves had been a container for the honouring of both life and death. This was a short programme of workshops, not therapy sessions, and therefore did not allow for deep and confidential sharing. Nevertheless, it seemed a useful starting place for people needing to process and reflect at a safe level whist enjoying and building the community spirit through shared art-making. It was

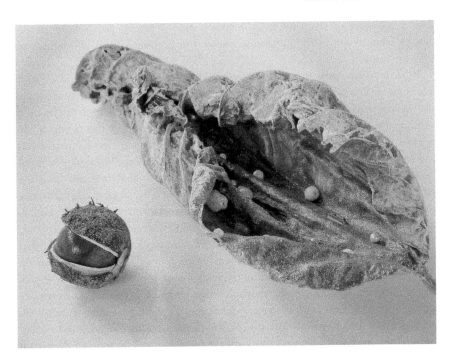

FIGURE 12.4   Leaf of death

an opportunity to share and honour the roots that they have grown from and the routes that their lives have taken. Usually in art therapy sessions I do not participate in the art-making. On this occasion it had felt an important part of the group process to accept the invitation to join in with the creativity. My own creation had helped to forge a powerful connection between some patients, staff and myself. The artwork had conveyed my empathic sentiments and the process of endings, where words failed me. The use of organic materials meant that the changing process from life to death could be communicated in a new way in the hospice. I was struck by the power of one leaf to represent the frailty and transience of life.

Embracing nature's cycles can help people develop flexibility, working with loss, uncertainty and unpredictability. Exploring different perspectives helps to develop coping mechanisms and resilience. The material offered from the natural environment can have a unique power to bring about conversations around lack of control, life, death and change. The workshops appeared to create a sensory opportunity which enabled people to take time to reflect, through the process of developing artwork that embodies both an individual's inner and outer world. In addition, outdoor materials are free, versatile and not harmful for the environment. The process takes people outside of their normal working and living space, either physically, psychologically or both. Nature calls for a playfulness that frees the inner child, marshalling our creative resources and inner strength. I have repeatedly observed how spending time in and with nature restores the connection to feeling, bypassing cognitive defence mechanisms, to aid recovery and self-healing. Environmental arts therapy takes us out of the institution, and our institutional selves, and returns us back to nature.

It came as no surprise that there was such a need for reflective and creative spaces for professionals who work in the hospice. Many shared that they continually shelved their feelings of being overwhelmed, distressed and burned out by their continued experience of working with loss, in order to meet the needs of the patients. The workshop sessions offered staff time to reflect, care for themselves and an opportunity to encourage one another. There was some ambivalence about these staff workshops, as it was considered a luxury to take time out from the patients and the many tasks needing to be carried out. Nevertheless, the staff spoke about how they would value a regular space to take care of their needs, an opportunity to discuss and process their feelings and build better rapport with each other.

It was clear that the need for positivity as a coping mechanism on the part of both the patients and the staff was serving to cover up the grieving process at the end of life and working creatively with nature proved to be a safe way of approaching this, albeit given the short time that we had together. This had felt like a powerful and at times vulnerable experience for us all. In a country so rich with storytelling, it had been an opportunity for participants to use wild and natural materials, themes and metaphors as a means of telling and honouring their own stories, as they confront the most wild and natural experience of all.

References

Fosztó, L. (2009). *Ritual revitalisation after socialism: Community, personhood, and conversion among Roma in a Transylvanian village*. New Brunswick: LIT Verlag.

Huet, V. (2017). Case study of an art therapy-based group for work-related stress with hospice staff. *International Journal of Art Therapy*, 22 (1), pp. 22–34.

Mosoiu, D., Andrews, C., and Perolls, G. (2000). Palliative care in Romania. *Palliative Medicine*, 14 (1), pp. 65–67.

Ncube, N., and Denborough, D. (2008). *The tree of life*. Retrieved from: https://dulwichcentre.com.au/the-tree-of-life/.

Teodorescu, A. (2015). *Death representations in literature: Forms and theories*. Newcastle Upon: Cambridge Scholars Publishing Tyne.

13

GROWING ELDERS

The cultivation and collaboration of an elder women's group in the woods

Deborah Kelly and Vanessa Jones

Introduction

This chapter explores the development of an elder women's group, working in and with nature, in woodland in the south of England. It is written from our perspective as facilitators *and* as elders ourselves, and thus resonates with ethnographic study as well as reflexive practice. The voice of the group participants is heard indirectly, through our considerations. Anonymized examples of the group experience are used occasionally to illustrate a point. We felt it important for the group members to read the work before publication, which they have done. Not only did we receive their permission but also their encouragement to share our findings. Comments from the group have been incorporated into the writing to ensure that it remains resonant with their experiences.

Roots

In its beginning years, the group was created for women therapists aged over fifty years old. We ran it as a closed therapeutic group, meeting for one day, eight times a year, in semi-private woodland. Initially, seven older women answered our call to work with what it might mean to live as aging women.

It was not a psychotherapy group with the purpose of exploring and transforming personal difficulty. Instead we hoped to create a space where the wood and her non-human inhabitants and elements would teach and support our exploration of living and dying as elders. In creating the group as arts psychotherapists our role, as we saw it, was to form the intention for the work, devise structure, hold space, keep time and offer the women participants different embodied, exploratory and creative arts therapy practices in the woodland. As facilitators we co-created the space from two different primary psychotherapy trainings and separate life experiences.

This created a rich dialogue and exchange of ideas between us culminating in some surprising developments. Although Vanessa has trained with Ian Siddons Heginworth, and therefore brought aspects of environmental arts therapy into the mix, this was never a purely environmental arts therapy group. We developed our own particular co-facilitation style together, drawing on a variety of approaches including imaginal, natural, embodied and psychotherapeutic roots.

Deborah

I came into the work from a health professional background, including training in both Western and Eastern medicine and body work. My interest in shiatsu, body energy, land energy and sacred landscapes brought me into working with nature as a teacher and then as an integrative arts psychotherapist. I use many creative media, visual and embodied, story and myth, deeply grounded in what Dawkins (1998) might call the work of love, for nature and the sacred lands. I am particularly interested in the therapeutic potential of place and pilgrimage, which for me can include the world of the imagination.

Vanessa

My background was as an artist, working in the UK and US exploring anthropological and sociopolitical ideas. As a performance artist I produced aesthetic, time-based public actions hoping to inspire change. This led to activism, then working in Africa for an NGO, before training as an arts therapist. I see clear links between this and the embodied ritual work we do in the woods. It also takes me into the public green spaces of the city where I work turning seemingly unpromising public land into treasured therapeutic landscapes (Jones et al., 2016).

On different paths, developing knowledge from separate specialisms and divergent contexts, we share an interest in research, nature and embodied imagination. We both fundamentally believe in the therapeutic potential of being in and with nature. There is a vast and growing amount of evidence of this; how it benefits our physical, mental and spiritual health and facilitates a reciprocal relationship, helping us to give ecological attention to the health of the Earth. Having experience of working within National Health Service (NHS) paradigms, we have both found our way into working within the healing potential of natural environments; a move outwards literally and into the world yet involving a deep re-membering of our belonging to nature and the cosmos; a coming home.

Beginning in 2012, we chose to run the Women Elders Group at or near the eight solar festivals. For us, this structure is inherent in the natural world. It is familiar and offers a way to meet at the turning of the seasons. Yet, more profoundly, we recognize these fire festivals as marking significant points in the rhythm of the Earth, celebrated over thousands of years by our ancestors. These full and cross quarter points were vital for connecting to and maintaining an interdependent relationship with the Earth, the gods and humankind, acting as power points in time and space. They provide a way for the group to re-connect with and explore the meaning, metaphors and stories within the wheel of the year, as well as to celebrate and renew the energy for the world (Dawkins, 1998; Siddons Heginworth, 2008). In terms of elderhood, they offer a form to examine and embrace the energy of all life from birth to the rising feminine energy of maiden and mother, the masculine energy of the sun and the decline of both into old age and stillness: Maiden, Mother, Crone; birth, death and rebirth.

Now in its fifth year (at the point of writing) the women's elder group has shifted its rhythm. No longer meeting eight times a year as a closed group, we meet four times a year at the Celtic cross quarter fire festivals, with an additional annual summer celebration camp. Our solstice and equinox meetings are now open sessions for adults of all ages, professions and genders, as well as for the established group. This organic process of change grew from a need to address questions of sustainability as a group, wanting to grow our numbers, yet grow in a way that opens diversity of membership and varied options for long-term or brief participation. For us it seemed to mirror something of both the constancy and variety of the seasons. The natural world through its long, long history, clearly shows that *not* to change can mean stagnation and death.

The story of the wood

The wood in which we work offers us a way to be with nature: an invitation to listen, remember, align ourselves in heart and soul to her rhythms and also to the rhythm of the wider Earth and the cosmos. The group uses shelter in the wood, alongside its natural spaces, in the form of a wooden hut, a yurt and a mud and wattle round house.

Set in the high weald in southern England, the mixed ancient woodland is surrounded by fields and stands on soft clay and sandstone from the Cretaceous Period. During the last ice age much of southern England resembled Arctic tundra, but as time passed and as the climate warmed the land became forested. As the land bridge between Britain and Europe was lost under the rising sea levels, trees that had already colonized became our native species. This one-hundred-acre wood, over time, has been cut for timber, dug for sandstone for building, mined for iron ore for smelting and provided charcoal for gunpowder and iron works. The surrounding fields have been grazed for sheep and cattle and supported grass and grain crops.

Today, the woodland is defined by its chestnut coppicing run on fifteen-year rotations. The seasons and the coppicing provide a rhythm to the woods changing the sounds, scents, colour and views as nature and man create different vistas. The feel of the wood changes too, through time, but also place. Some areas are left to nature, some are tangled and boggy, others more spacious, scented and dry. There are areas of high ground and valleys, public walks and quiet, private places. Different trees, ancient and new, cast their shadows and roots onto and into the land. Some are dying. The chestnut and ash are under threat from imported diseases (carried on the wind or by commercial plants). Yet Nature herself seems to thrive here, in spite of this.

The woodland has been host to various groups over decades, from ecotherapists and shamanic practitioners, to yoga groups, shiatsu workshops and gestalt group therapy. There have been forest schools for children, camping programmes for teenagers, weddings, drumming groups, sweat lodges, men's groups, palliative care groups and burials.

We have come to see the flow of land workers, practitioners, past group participants and friends as quietly working and enriching the soil over the decades and creating pathways through the trees, deepening the sense of place, as 'song lines' of the wood. Sometimes we walk in harmony, sometimes counterpoint, to past footsteps and intentions.

Therapeutic potential

All the natural elements of the wood provided teachings: the quality of a tree, the wildlife and fauna, the turning of time, the sensuality of the place, the spontaneous moments or created acts unfolding before us. We drew on all of this facilitating within the frame of arts psychotherapy. Yet we also worked with space and land energy, extending the therapeutic potential beyond the familiar frame towards a collaboration with the wisdom of the trees and the land, the animals and stories of the ancestors.

Over the years, at significant points in the wheel of the year, we have offered sacred walks and mini pilgrimages, labyrinth and spiral work, meditative, embodied and contemplative group experiences; we have enacted the myths resonant with the seasons. We made time to rest, listening deeply to the way of nature in the wood, developing a receptivity to the wood as teacher and guide. We moved into creative acts with found material. A rhythm developed in the work embracing shared time and creative process, individual experiences, check ins and check outs. We shared around what one participant calls the 'living fire' at the centre of our circle: a candle lit bowl in the yurt, the open wood fire within the wood. The importance of a 'potluck' lunch became a rich reflection of nature's bounty – a place to bring, share and celebrate our own (and our family's) culinary, pickling and gardening wisdom and heritage. These meals were also a time to talk in the everyday language of elders.

Why elder womanhood?

The idea of an elder women's group held many layers for us to explore both as practitioners and as elders ourselves. We started from where we were – aging women, in aging bodies, reclaiming and exploring that identity first. Participants told their personal sacred story of menstruation through to menopause, resonant with ideas drawn from the red tent movement and the work of Alexandra Pope (2013). We honoured the natural wisdom of the womb, our feminine cycles of fertility and of course the natural movement towards death. We wanted to explore what it felt like to grow old consciously and as a group.

We drew on myth, poetry and song from a great lineage of female writers, artists, healers and wise women, such as Sharon Blackie (2016), Carolyn Hillyer (2010),

Clarissa Pinkola Estes (2008) and Marion Woodman (1985). Yet not only women writers informed or intrigued us. We were drawn to the imaginal and beauty within nature (Abram, 1997; Corbin, 1989; May, 1985; Hillman, 1975) and a curiosity to explore the wholeness of psyche beyond our womanhood.

We were aware of a paradox around the focus on women and gender and a potential resistance to restrict or be separatist. We preferred to think of all things as containing both yin and yang principles. Yet as we grow older we notice the particularity of aging as a woman, a time when 'femininity' is fading in a physical sense as our oestrogen declines. The loss of fertility and the changes in our bodies are peculiar to our *female* bodies even though our sensibilities may embrace all the fluidity within gender and sexuality.

Perhaps that is why we are drawn as facilitators and elder women to Mother Earth. As our aging bodies stop their cycles of menstruation, it may be that as crones we are learning to navigate and synchronise with the slower, everlasting deep rhythm of the universe – the movement of the celestial bodies. Our ritual and ceremony together mark particular gateways in the passage of time and offer ways to connect collectively as elders with the great mother Gaia, celebrating the larger feminine cycle of birth, death and rebirth, towards a wider rhythm of the cosmos.

Another paradox arises in our thinking about elderhood as 'wise' in an aging population. Arguably, the designation of 'wise elder' in past times was assigned to those who had managed to defy the will of death into an old age. These people were unusual in reaching such an age and as such were revered and respected. Now we, as elders, are the norm, a power to be captured (the grey vote, the silver surfers) or a potential drain on society, health care and family. Could this sense of decline and social burden be another reason that as elder women we turn back towards Mother Earth to try to reclaim our femininity and power? After all, what is greater and more constant than the Earth? Even the sun diminishes each day for half the year.

This reclamation of power and wisdom can be seen through the frame of a 56-year cycle as Dawkins (1998) proposes, superimposed on the wheel of the year. He explains that if the passage between each of the eight solar festivals represents seven years of our lives, and we are born at the winter solstice, then we reach puberty at spring (aged 14), intellectual height at 28 (the summer solstice), and we lose our fertility at All Hallows as the year declines. The winter solstice brings us to a metaphorical death at age 56. With the very real potential now to live through two cycles, the second cycle brings us to a new awakening, a rebirth as 'grandmothers' with the opportunity to experience the circle again, at least in part. We recapture the rising maiden and mother energy of spring and summer once more, but this time perhaps with a wiser and wider view. We take our life out into the world as teachers, elders, grandmothers, as we move towards our physical death. Within this frame, old age is no longer seen merely as decline but as a richer life, a deepening into soul in service to the world.

The concept of 'grandmother' came naturally into the elder group as a way of being, and more archetypally as a personal support to each participant. In the group's beginning each elder was invited to find her 'grandmother tree': a particular tree that drew her, to become for her the essence of grandmothering. These trees were revisited on each meeting and the relationship between woman and tree deepened and expanded over time. The tree of course was just a tree, *and* it was a grandmother tree that could be rested on, listened to, meditated under, leaned on and dreamed with. Our initial purpose was to facilitate the creation of a secure base for each group member. As such, we could ensure this tree was not going to be cut down. Yet our relationship to the trees required us to acknowledge the

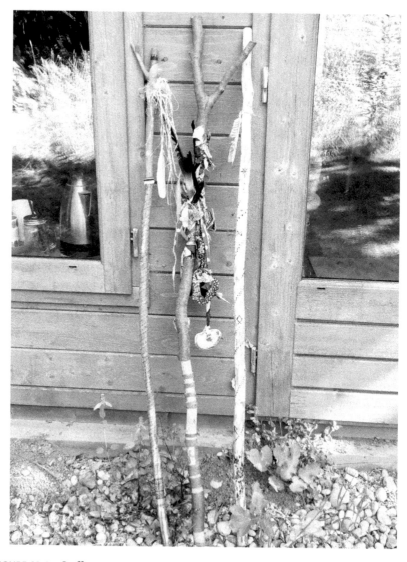

FIGURE 13.1 Staffs

impermanence within nature. Our trees were subject to storms, damage and death just as we were. Somehow though, each tree became a rooted, steady, benign and wise presence for each participant as our group progressed.

We also asked the wood to offer us physical support. As a gentle initiation into the group and into the wood, each elder created a staff from hazel or rowan, to peel and carve and decorate, to act as a support and as a symbol of her travels (Figure 13.1). This was a beautiful individual process that continued over the years, the staffs often becoming part of the rituals and the subject of some lighthearted staff envy! Perhaps this resonates with various cultural symbolism and myths where the staff represents a masculine energy. For example, the axis mundi rises through the feminine earth; the staff of Asclepius is entwined with the snake of earth wisdom and healing. The staffs became works of art as well as imbued with symbolic meaning and practical use for aging bodies, a weaving together of nature and woman and of yin and yang.

Facilitation

Initially we presented a facilitation style that incorporated a planned structure including a check in, group experience, feedback and reflective process. Whilst holding appropriate professional boundaries, we remained open and adaptive to what might emerge from the experience of the group.

As we grew towards a familiarity with each other, the participants, the land and the changing seasons, we allowed the days to evolve inviting creative exploration, research and discovery in a more fluid way. As time went on, we noticed a difference developing from our usual therapeutic practice – a shift of focus towards a kind of 'unknowing'.

In some ways it meant we did less as facilitators, as the wood and the world of imagination were engaged with and embraced. In other ways, and perhaps because the focus resonated with us too, we found ourselves experimenting with boundaries within and without ourselves. Sometimes we shared in a ritual, or exercise, exploring the potential for our own participation. Thus, our professional boundaries extended to a holding and a belonging: one foot outside the circle, one-foot in. Sometimes this was done with one of us fully participating, such as experiencing an intuitive walk, while the other held the space. Sometimes we both joined in a ritual, yet mindful of a facilitative energy that held the experience lightly yet clearly.

The freedom, lightness and intuitive sense of this developed further as the group relationships deepened and an understanding of our role as facilitators, as women and as elders was experienced, reflected on, and practiced.

Deeper and deeper

As we explored the wood and her surrounding land more deeply over the years we all became more attuned to the natural energy in the landscapes, inspiring different emotional, physical, even spiritual experiences. We experienced different times and weather through night walks, morning breezes, stillness and wild winds.

We noticed too, how perspectives changed depending on which story we were 'inside' and in which place or season. For example, inside the story of our decline and dying, we might see and feel disease in nature: the crooked branch, the broken limb, the steep incline on a walk, the autumn leaves falling as they fade and dry. Or we might see beauty everywhere as time becomes more precious (Figure 13.2). Our felt experiences in spring, or in an open field, may evoke a longing for youth

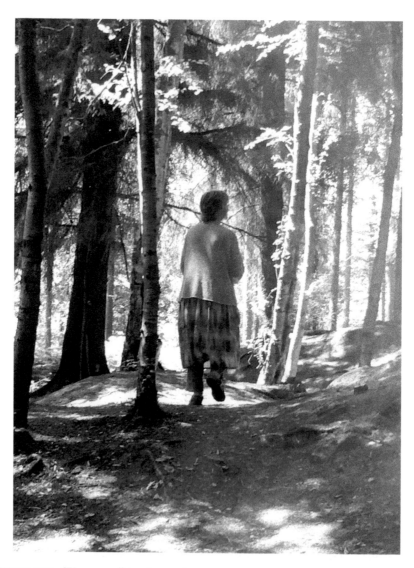

FIGURE 13.2 Woman walking in woods

and expansion or a celebration of freedom as we age. The wood, the elements and the land thus played their own part in the groups' experience.

Sacred places

Whilst nature provided different landscapes – some healing, some challenging – we also created therapeutic and sacred spaces through ritual and ceremony in small and large ways. As Eliade writes (1987), the repetitive nature of ritual celebration adds power and strength to the work and to all who have done these rituals before and will do again. Moving from the profane to the sacred and working with intention, we considered that this deep work could be transformative on many levels, bringing us away from individual acts, towards community.

However, nature also offered her spontaneous power to transform with no devised preparation, except perhaps a growing openness within the group, to moments of epiphany (Jauregui, 2007). We were blessed with beauty or moments of synchronicity and power that gave us deep experiences often beyond words. For example, on a night walk we planned to rest in the twilight of the day and explore the question of the twilight of our life. As we entered the field which gave us the clearest view of the evening sky, the place filled with bright mist so enthralling and unexpected it left us breathless. One by one we walked silently into the mist as if into another world and lay down in the wet grass, lost and invisible to the world we had left. It was experienced that evening as a practice for death, only this time we could return into the clear night. Nature had facilitated a profound experience and each emerged transformed.

This was no planned or prepared ritual but rather a gift. Each person entering the mist seemed open to such miracles prepared perhaps in some other way. We were learning to follow where the wood leads, to engage in the changing energy of the land, to embrace these moments of deep meaning without the need to rationalize them out of existence, and we felt the richer for it.

Moving outwards

From these and many more sacred experiences, we developed the concept that our 'work' in the woods as an elder group might somehow flow out to the wider world, either literally through our own communities or through ritual into the 'world soul' (Hillman, 1975). Marie Geneen Haugen's (2013) description of her daily ritual of flute playing for the land is an example of a sacred act flowing outwards. She understands it as a participation with the natural world – a participation that is needed, that matters. Our hope, too, was that we could explore elderhood in service of a wider and broader potential beyond individual self-awareness.

This development of the group coincided with a change in facilitation style. Our approach opened further trusting in the power and mystery of the wood, trusting imagination, psyche and nature to play their part. Having created the space, we learned to get out of the way.

As time went on we continued to hold a vision of therapeutic exploration that flowed from the inner 'I' towards collaboration and outwards to the world. In the first two years we had moved from individual creative and embodied exploration of elderhood in the group (I) to holding space for the group of elders (We) before gradually embracing a broader and deeper consciousness of a group in service of the world (All).

This movement outwards provoked practical changes. Rather than offering a series of deepening exercises as we did in the early years, concluding the day with verbal reflective process at the fireside, we now simply set a planned intention for each session. Lightly and intuitively we stepped out from there, gathering stories, images and experiences which would form a closing ritual or ceremonial embodying all action created by the group, mindful of and with intention for the wider community and the Earth. This 'in service for the world' can also be seen from a more transpersonal or shamanic perspective. Alongside belief in the power of prayer and ritual – of Earth pilgrimage, of walking with love – we consider that individual acts may have universal influence. We do not consider this inflated, but linked to the potential work of an elder, to take our learning back into the world *in service* of others. From another perspective it was a simple acknowledgment that we are connected to everything, that the universal is in the particular (Braud, 1997) and each act, like the beat of a butterfly's wings, has an influence on the world. This resonates perhaps with Johnstone and Macy's writing (2012) where the idea of a shared intelligence and visionary impulses are seen as "accessing the wisdom of the whole on behalf of the whole" (Johnstone and Macy, 2012, p. 176).

We were moving from more traditional frames of psychotherapy; continuing to think as psychotherapists yet also leaning into broader systemic frames such as described in Gregory Bateson's *A Sacred Unity* (1991) and his daughter Cathy Bateson's work in cybernetics. Here both practitioners remind us that being human starts in unison, in utero, and that it is primarily only the west which promotes the separate, all-powerful individual. They describe 'the illusion of independence' growing from the quest for individual power, away from natural relationship with mother, families, peoples and the Earth – a position of connectedness and inter-dependency.

Most recently we have developed our facilitation style further, inviting the stories of individual encounters, dreams, and artworks or felt bodily experience to be returned to the group in metaphor, as story or poetry rather than rationalized. We began experimenting with removing personal reflection and processing which can take us out of contact with each other and with the experience. We were curious to remain 'in the dream making all day', where we may stay aligned to something more than individual awareness. This proved an extraordinary deepening of the work. In this way the women's words are accepted into the therapeutic space to be transmuted and/or returned to the wood and the world. Self-regulation, if needed, came through community, embodiment and the earth. The wood held the space. There was no need for the therapeutic processing that we usually considered essential. The change had happened. The 'work' was contained by the wood, the ancestors, the community of elders and we were transformed.

These words provide an example of group poetic 'feedback' after a reflective exercise in the wood.

> *Holding elderhood in mind,*
> *I lost myself in the air*
> *And in the air*
> *and in the tops of the trees*
> *And in song*
> *I felt the roots go down*
> *into something alive*
>
> *And holding elderhood in mind,*
> *humming and vibrating*
> *I felt myself go up*
> *into something humming and vibrating*
> *with the hoverflies and the trees*
> *and us and the roots*
> *and I stayed in one place*
> *and yet I was everywhere*
>
> *I am reminded of fruitfulness*
> *I am reminded of the cyclical rise and fall*
> *And the constant freedom of both*
>
> *I put my ear to the ground*
> *and heard the deafening roar of history*
> *And I grieve for the land that I left*
> *The dirt that I left*
>
> *I embrace ancientness*
>
> *I remember my grandmother tree*
> *Memory held in the wood*
> *More reliably than memory*
>
> *I feel tired*
> *and like I'm just beginning*

And later, after the group, one participant sends further writing:

Black dog and buzzard call

> *The fire, intended to be just a small beacon rears up*
> *The sisters, a group of love plunder the shadows*

Light hints at dark and flickers in the heat which burns us
It is all here
The hoverflies suspended, hum their constant vibration
The understory, insistent and tetchy, trembles and darts off
A black dog thunders through our space and vanishes
It is all here
Bluebeards blood appears as a blackcurrant stain
Pavlova and syllabub spread and mark us
Tears fall as brothers ride over the horizon
It is all here
Buzzards call to us, fecund red bugs perform their
Consummation
Cow parsley decays, scent hangs intense
Dragonflies create questions for us
It is all here
Memories of magic gone before, comes back to claim us
Hares, owls, tigers and creatures cry
A truth mandala imprint in the retina
Predators and princesses locked up
Destruction spun through life, death laced with potency, hate
Twisted with love
Longing and loss woven into our nature
We have an opportunity to choose to look closely and to see
More and ever more.

By Laura Jacobs (group participant)

In this way, our experience is reflected on as poetry and later reflected back through creative responses from the day, from our individual and collective experience. Through continued connection in between meetings via technology the work engenders ripples of discovery and knowing, iterative waves of inquiry and imagery – a call, a response and an emerging responsibility to the continuation of our work outside the meetings.

So, we share our learning and experiences, much as a training group might, through an email group continuing to explore themes, cross fertilizing ideas, sharing recipes and information, sending images, photographs and poems, creative pieces made in the continuation of personal and group experience. These shared communications weave together cyber links to websites, artists, political acts, literature and research, supporting the group to continue in the 'widening circles' (Rilke, 1905) described as enriching the cauldron of learning and in reciprocity with one another and the Earth. In short, we see the genesis of a small outward flow ensuring the continuity of practices and discovery into the world and our living beyond the wood.

Reflections on the work as elders

We discover that the deeper we go, the wider we travel. As we hold the triple goddess as an archetypal and mythic energy calling us together, we also celebrate each person's uniqueness, embracing the diversity within our stories and songs. Nature shows us the way in this, through the ever-changing web of life, emerging constantly from the exquisite beauty of individual threads.

. . . on being in the world as elders

Humour has been a frequent companion within our growing elderhood, sometimes as ribald laughter or the simple comedy of our aging bodies, sap rising nevertheless. "*Laughter*", one participant commented, "*is part of our medicine, part of the mix, transcending and transforming the elements we cook . . . around the fire.*"

Yet the fireside sharing also turned towards more serious concerns. Around the fire and over lunch the women discussed the troubles that continue to take place in their own, in their loved one's lives and in the lives of others far outside the wood.

In its first five years the group has lived through significant sociopolitical shocks. There has been a Brexit referendum in the UK. Worldwide we have seen the corruption of democratic elections and the rise of authoritarian leaders. As the years went by the list of inter-racial, inter-faith and inter-gender conflict, oppression and injustice seemed to spread, alongside the growing environmental exigencies.

There is an old story we sometimes use, retold by Carolyn Baker (Baker, 2011, pp. 157–158), of an old woman weaving an exquisite cloth in the darkness of her cave. She stops only occasionally to stir her cooking pot at the other end of cave, attending to a soup made of all that is good in the world, lest it should burn and spoil. As she does this, and each time she does this, her black crow comes and unravels all her exquisite weaving. The elder returns from the cooking pot and picks up her cloth reweaving the change without complaint – for what is life but the picking up and the recreating from all the trouble in our own and our children's lives?

Typically, within psychotherapy the tapestries we weave are based on the singular 'I' threads, or at least the human story, where disruption and trouble are the focus of change. But the story of the crone in the cave teaches us that the interruptions and trouble are attended to by the elder for the world, not for the 'I'. These are the threads that she picks up and works with even when undone, to weave the cloth into order and beauty again. She is rather like nature, perhaps indifferent to our struggles, just picking up after breaking down and stirring with the persistence and intention of Physis – the Protogenoi goddess of life, fertility, weather and natural forces – to maintain the soup of 'all that is good in the world'.

Whilst it may burn in our bones to see oppression and suffering, the wood teaches us that while humans may drive themselves into extinction, nature, like the crone, will likely adapt and continue through our unraveling. Our grandmother trees teach us of rootedness and solidity. As we have noted the group's creative and imaginal work has become an act of service, a gesture into the world and for the world like the crone in the cave, yet borne from a deep sympathy with all things, a *sumpatheia ton hollon* (Moriarty, 2009). Our practice in the wood, to remember our belonging, might now stand as a root to our activism, taking the form of quiet ritual as well as public marches – rituals of intention, acts of meditation, ways of being. This way our actions as elders, whether silent or loud, might contain the stillness and power of the tree, the patience and persistence of the crone.

. . . on resource and reciprocity as elders

Within ecotherapy, we find that the notion of nature as a 'resource' to be used and exploited is condemned. Yet if we hyphenate the word 'resource', we discover that we can re-source ourselves, not by using up limited resources from the Earth, but simply by coming back to the idea that we are part of nature. It is not that we are working *in* nature but that we are already part of it. There is a flow of energy which can be there for us and all nature to tap into, belong to, give thanks for, rather than use up or exploit. Thus comes reciprocity.

We are using nature's resource to re-source and restore ourselves and we are offering something back to the wood: our warmth, our attention, our imagination and our praise. We maintain reciprocity through ritual thanks and creative acts, but also by ensuring the regeneration of the wood. As we learn from the wood, from one another and the world, we grow our group as a reciprocal act. So that gradually our footsteps may deepen in love for the Earth and eventually, as elders, we will give back our bodies to the earth.

. . . as death approaches in our elderhood

The wood invites us in our elderhood to reconnect with the Earth and life, but as we come towards our dying and our death, the wood can teach us about this too. Death must happen to engender life. We see this simply in the changing seasons: in the fox that kills a rabbit to feed her cubs, in leaves falling to feed the soil. Whilst a single tree may die the wood continues and so we get glimpses of something eternal and our place in the natural cycle of things. Whilst wild nature may not suffer the existential angst of humans that feeds our fear of death and decline, it can teach us the natural necessity of death and the impermanence of our individuality. As the earth calls for our returning and nature invites us to consider time beyond our comprehension, we see our lives in true perspective (Kelly, 2016).

Our work with imagination, sacred space and ritual also teaches us to cross thresholds into other worlds, into the *mundus imaginalis* (Corbin, 1989), a practice which some have described as preparations for death (Grof, n.d.; Strong, 2005). One autumn we invited the group to experience leaf burials, each carving out and clearing a place on the earth where she would be buried. Another group member then buried her in leaves where she remained to contemplate her death. Creatures crawled over each body and into the leaves and the wind blew as they dropped into reverie. One wrote:

> As I grew still, I felt as though I were being forgotten by nature – forgotten as a human, as a separate thing, but remembered and claimed as part of the wood, my body dissolving into the leaves. I felt more than me, a sense of completeness as 'I' diminished.

As a maiden with life ahead of her, there is potential to activate change and to see the change; as a mother we consider the place in which our children grow, looking towards their future. As an old woman, a crone, we must consider the world as we leave it behind. Yet we may also sense this diminishing boundary as the earth reclaims us. We can teach our children and grandchildren that death is part of nature, and that we all belong to the eternal part of life that remains: the earth, the stars, the sea and the mountains.

Summary

Our reflections have led us to consider the place this work has in psychotherapy and specifically arts and environmental arts therapy from the perspective of elder practitioners.

Each elder participant is a part of a collaborative therapeutic agency and presence, experiencing and working with nature, imagination, the group, community, history, story and ancestors. For those aspects to be alive and present, for their wisdom to be felt, we as facilitators need to 'get out of the way', to create a space or structure simply to hold the unfolding experience. We place our trust in that, rather than in any particular theoretical technique or intervention.

So have we moved away from our therapeutic roots? We think not. Our roots remain in the soil of our training and experience of life. Yet we have developed a few more branches that seem to be drawn towards a more collaborative and intuitive vision of therapeutic potential. The 'therapeutic relationship' is no longer confined to practitioner and client or even the triadic relationship with the art image (Schaverien, 1999). It is much wider than that, reminding us that we are part of the world and part of nature capable of exploring and experiencing our lives and the world in multiple ways and relationships.

Partnership, collaboration and community engender a different practice model from our original psychotherapy trainings. It is neither individual therapeutic process nor group process – it is more than these. Perhaps it is more akin to social change or art. It includes environmental arts therapy teaching, integrative arts therapy and meditative creativity, rather than ecotherapy or psychotherapy in woods. But it is not intended as art, environmental or social activism. We bring these in, yet we also see, simply, a growing band of wild elders cooking nourishing organic full-bodied fruitiness. Participants have described the work as *expanding, inspiring and life giving*, not just for each elder but with our active hope, perhaps, for the world too.

At times our eldering flowers, at other times we vanish into the mists, becoming part of the flow of this powerful place and of all nature. Like the old crone in the cave, this group's work is also, simply, to work the threads of our living here, and learning together with the wood how we might prepare for death.

The group deepens and goes on, widening its circle sometimes, then reducing in number, then widening again. We have grown with these expansions and contractions, each wave a creative opportunity. We could not know that this group would become as it is now. The fact is it has been continuing on through times of threatened extinction and still with each cycle it seems to re-form in unexpected ways; it returns again more wild and beautiful. Perhaps this is how both the wood and the Earth of which she is a part feel, too. When we allow Physis her power, when we go with her deeper into the anima mundi and stay open to what may be revealed, we may encounter miracles.

References

Abram, D. (1997). *The spell of the sensuous*. New York: Vintage.

Baker, C. (2011). *Navigating the coming chaos: A handbook for inner transition*. New York: iUniverse Inc.

Bateson, G. (1991). *A sacred unity: Further steps to an ecology of mind*. London: Harper Collins.

Blackie, S. (2016). *If women rose rooted. The journey to authenticity and belonging*. Tewkesbury: September Publishing.

Braud, W. (1997). *The ley and the labyrinth: Universalistic and particularistic approaches to knowing*. Retrieved from: https://static.secure.website/wscfus/326656/uploads/LeyAndLabyrinth.pdf.

Corbin, H. (1989). *Spiritual body and celestial earth*. Princeton: Princeton University Press.

Dawkins, P. (1998). *Zoence, the science of life*. Maine: Samuel Weiser.

Eliade, M. (1987). *The sacred and profane: The nature of religion*. Orlando, FL: Harcourt.

Grof, S. (n.d.). *The experience of death and dying: Psychological, philosophical and spiritual aspects* [Online]. Retrieved from: http//www.stanislavgrof.com/wpcontent/upload.

Haugen, M.G. (2013). Imagining earth. In Vaughan-Lee, Llewellyn (Ed.), *Spiritual ecology: The cry of the earth* (pp. 159–171). Point Reyes, CA: The Golden Sufi Centre.

Hillman, J. (1975). *Revisioning psychology*. New York: Harper and Row.

Hillyer, C. (2010). *Sacred house: Where women weave words into the earth*. Postbridge, Devon: Seventh Wave Books.

Jauregui, A. (2007). *Epiphanies: Where science and miracles meet*. New York: Atria Books.

Johnstone, C., and Macy, J. (2012). *Active hope: How to face the mess we're in without going crazy*. Novato, CA: New World Library.

Jones, V., Thompson, B., and Watson, J. (2016). Feet on the ground and branching out. In Jordan, M., and Hinds, J. (Eds.), *Ecotherapy: Theory research and practice* (pp. 162–175). London: Palgrave.

Kelly, D. (2016). Working with nature in palliative care. In Jordan, M., and Hinds, J. (Eds.), *Ecotherapy: Theory research and practice* (pp. 84–94). London: Palgrave.

May, R. (1985). *My quest for beauty*. Dallas, TX: Saybrook Publishing.

Moriarty, J. (2009). *Dreamtime*. Dublin: The Lilliput Press.

Pinkola–Estes, C. (2008). *Women who run with the wolves*. London: Rider.

Pope, A. (2013). *The woman's quest: Unfolding women's path of power and wisdom*. London: New Generation Publishing.

Rilke, R.M. (1905). *Rilke's book of hours. Love poems to god*. Translated by Burrows, A., and Macy, J. (2005). New York: Riverhead Books.

Schaverien, J. (1999). *The revealing image*. London: Jessica Kingsley.

Siddons Heginworth, I. (2008). *Environmental arts therapy and the tree of life*. Exeter: Spirit Rest.

Strong, L. (2005). *Psychopomp stories: Contemplating death in a spiritually diverse society*. Doctoral Dissertation, Pacifica Graduate Institute (Unpublished). Retrieved from: https://pre.hsls.pitt.edu/medical-humanities-dissertations/all?topic . . . month=2007/03.

Woodman, M. (1985). *The pregnant virgin*. Toronto: Inner City Books.

EPILOGUE

Ian Siddons Heginworth

Whenever we walk the wild road on, whether in life or in death, we cannot know what lies beyond. All that we can be sure of is that everything is about to change.

We live in a remarkable time. A time when a teenage girl can walk out of her school in Sweden to protest about governmental inaction in response to climate change, and within a matter of months millions of students and school children all over the world are following her example and doing the same on a monthly basis. Only the internet and social media could allow this to happen. So it is that the thing which we as parents most often fear might alienate our children from their relationship with nature now becomes the very tool that they use in their quest to reclaim it.

This uprising of the children gives me so much hope, because the voice of the child is the voice of the heart. The heart knows inherently when something is wrong. When the children take to the streets they make this voice heard at last above the clamour of our intellectual excuse making, and our own hearts recognising the truth in their words, are moved to act.

Of course, the obstacles are as vast as the odds against us. We are all in the sway of an unrestrained masculine that cannot see beyond its own paradigm, that treats economic growth and technological progress as its holy grail to be pursued and fought for at all costs, even at the cost of the Earth. It is driven as much by its own relentless inertia as it is by fossil fuels; and the more we challenge it, the harder it will fight for its right to rule. But there is a new paradigm emerging, an uprising of the feminine alongside the welling up of the waters. In the words of one young man speaking at a climate rally in my own town, "The biggest grassroots movement the world has ever seen, since grass."

My generation grew up in a time when the feeling truth of a child was of little account. The use of physical violence as punishment was the norm, and sexual abuse was unacknowledged and shrouded in secrecy. Many children were sent away from their families to boarding school, some as young as seven, but even for those that were not, schools were often harsh and aggressive environments where vulnerability attracted only further abuse. Feeling was seen as weakness and only academic achievement, competition and status had value. The only way to survive was to close the heart.

In environmental arts therapy, so many of my clients bring these stories into the woods in order to work with these cruel legacies. Slowly, and with great tenderness, the wounded child is gathered from a place of shame and self-neglect and brought into the light to be honoured and cherished at last. That which was profaned is made sacred.

It is for this reason that environmental arts therapy, indeed all nature-based therapies, have such an important part to play in these remarkable times. People come into therapy because they are stuck. Stuck in repetitive and dysfunctional relationship patterns. Stuck in addictive or self-harmful behaviour. Stuck in depression, in anxiety or in shame. They are stuck because life is not linear, it is cyclical and every cycle requires emotional release to complete. Without letting go, there is no moving on. But if the heart is closed, how can we do this?

In environmental arts therapy we learn to move towards feeling not away from it. Active grieving becomes a practice for life and by aligning our own cycles with those of nature we learn that we are held and that all we are is welcome. All of this is done within nature, using her gifts, her wild and beautiful locations and her synchronistic teaching, and so as we learn to feel ourselves we feel her too, unfolding and changing within us. No longer are we simply walking through the woods. We are the woods.

This is perhaps the greatest teaching of all. As long as the contemporary paradigm portrays us as separate from nature then it easy to see ourselves as a cancer eating away at the body of the Earth, preventing her self-regulating systems from working, a deadly parasite bringing its host to their knees. But once we claim our birthright as a child of nature, once we truly feel ourselves as an essential part of her mysterious web, then we open up the possibility that we ourselves can be the self-regulating system that she needs most at this time. That the transformation of human consciousness is the cutting edge of ecological change and recovery.

The relationship between personal grief and ecological grief is raw and immediate. In four million years of hominid evolution, nothing has prepared us for this. We have no genetic memory upon which to draw in order to find an authentic feeling response to the collapse of the Earth's ecosystems. For all the generations that have come before us she was the ever enduring constant, the bedrock of our being. Is it any wonder that we find ourselves now paralysed like rabbits in the headlights of a speeding truck?

But fear is the gateway to grief. It sits on top like a frozen crust and when in therapy we break through we find below the strata of feelings that make up the mystery of our heart's truth. This is as true for our grief about the death of nature as for anything that we have loved and lost. As we work down through the strata, speaking our grief to the Earth or to our children, releasing and honouring our guilt, our shame, our anger and our sadness we come at last to love – the heart of the matter.

Here we begin to understand at last what it is that we must do, what is our own very personal contribution in these remarkable times. From the place of love, our love for the green Earth, our love for the other-than-human souls who inhabit it and our love for the children and grandchildren who will inherit it from us, we find the will and the courage to act.

INDEX

Page numbers in *italics* indicate figures and in **bold** indicate tables on the corresponding pages.

abuse 37, 50, 52, 117–118, 214; trust after 83
abusive mothers 80–83
active partner, nature as 36, 50, 58
adventure therapy 170
aesthetic distance 95, 110, 117
affect regulation 37
Alban Eiler 158
amygdala 53
anger, therapeutic release of 10
Antcliff, L. R. 53
anxiety, Mind in the City workshops on 161, 162
Art as Medicine 29
art therapy outdoors 11, 13–14; in adult mental health services (*see* mental health services, outdoor art therapy in adult); Celtic Ogham tree calendar 17–18, 124, 146; challenges and opportunities when moving 34–35; decentering in 144–145; emotional geographies and 138–139; Five Ways to Wellbeing model and 152–153; innovation in groupwork for 40; moving 142–145, *144*; Natursense 21; Outdoor Music Therapy (OdMT) 31–32; urban spaces and 139–141; Wild Things project 21; *see also* Bringing the Outside In; Circle of Trees groups; COATS (Community Outdoor Art Therapy Service); EarthWays; environmental arts therapy; turning year cycle outdoor art therapy

Art Therapy Outdoors (ATO)/pilot project (ATO.pp) 168, 172–173; co-facilitating and occupational therapy outdoors in 175; locations and experiences 173–174; outcomes and group processes in 175; referrals and risk assessment in 173; transportation and evaluation 174–175
assessment, risk and benefit 39–40, 171, 173, 178
Atkins, S. 29, 33, 40
attachment, secure 56–57
attachment-informed environmental arts therapy 61–62; body and emotion in 64–65; empathic identification and expansion of the self in 73–74, *75*; encounter in 66–68; flow of feeling in 65–66; love, attachment and loss and need for 62–64; mindfulness, mentalisation, meta-awareness and reflection in 71–73; play in 66, 68–70; returning to the field with another perspective in 75–76; ritual and myth in 66, 70–71
attention-deficit-disorder 37
autonomic nervous system (ANS) 53, 99
Autumn season 142; Mind in the City workshops 160, 161–162
aware walking 31

Baker, C. 67, 209
Banks, S. 73
Barrows, A. 49, 57
Bateson, C. 206
Bateson, G. 206
beauty 89, 148; of leaf of death 193–196, *194, 195*
"being alone together" 170
being in the world as elders 209–210
Belonging 82
belonging, feelings of 56–58, 122
Beltane festival 18
Berger, R. 32, 36, 37, 41, 138
Bion, W. 171
biophilic locus 52
Blackie, S. 200
Blakeman, V. 163
bodily based emotions 52
body and emotion in attachment-informed environmental arts therapy 64–65
body-mind connection 37
Book of Lecan, The 17
boundaries, therapeutic 34–35, 167
Bowlby, J. 56, 63
brain: autonomic nervous system (ANS) 53, 99; development of 52; neuro-biological synchronisation and 56
Brazier, C. 38, 40
breakdowns 122
Bringing the Outside In: abusive mother, inner tyrant and being unable to change explored in 80–83; Gaia as good enough mother and learning to mother ourselves in 86–87; group feedback on 87–89; introduction to 79–80; only knowing the wound in 83–86; trust and putting down roots in 83
Brown, M. 73
Brown, S. 69
Buzzell, L. 170

Cadwaladr, B. 167
Campbell, J. 71, 107, 116
Cartesian mind-body split 48
Casson, J. 117, 170
Celtic Ogham tree calendar 17–18, 34, 123–124, 146
Celtic Tree Oracle: A System of Divination, The 17
Celtic year 12
Celtic Yule celebration 155–156
Centre for Well-being 153
Chalquist, C. 170
Chesner, A. 110
Child in matchbox *13*

children: attachment in 56–57, 63–64; brain development in 52; co-dependency with mothers 81–82; connection and belonging felt by 56–58; effects of nature on development of 37; guns, bridges and portals in art therapy with 55–56; introduction to art therapy with 47–48; more-than-human nature in 48–50; mothers and (*see* Bringing the Outside In); nature inspiring imagination in 55; nature mask with 50–51, *51*; wild Amazonian man and 54–55
Christian iconography, suppressed feminine in 88
chronic fatigue/myalgic encephalomyelitis (CFS/ME): ascent from 101–102; case study inquiry into 94; conclusions on 102–104; encountering the wounded feminine in treating 100–101; introduction to 93–94; letting go of suppressed feelings in treating 97–99; resourcing for 96–97
Circle of Trees groups 17–18, 25; closing the circle in 149; edges of therapeutic encounters in nature with 148–149; emotional geographies and 139; indoors and outdoors and 140–141; introduction to 137–138; moving art therapy outdoors and 142–145, *144*; natural materials and metaphors in 145–146; natural spaces and 138–139; opening circle 140, *141*; physicality of body and earth and 141–142; urban spaces and 139–141
client safety 39
clinical space: safety of 34; stepping outside the 35
COATS (Community Outdoor Art Therapy Service): Autumn and 154–155, *156–157*; introduction to 151–153; Maryon Park community gardens and 163–164, *165*; Mind in the City workshops and 159–163; Spring and 158; Studio Upstairs and 153–154, 159; Summer and 159; Winter and 155–157
co-dependency in mothering 81–82
co-facilitating and occupational therapy outdoors 175
Cohen, G. 73
Community Environmental Arts Therapy (CEAT)/pilot project (CEAT.pp) 168; development of 168, 175–178; evaluation in 178; outcomes, experiences and creative processes in 178–180; referrals and risk assessments in 178

Community Mental Health Team (CMHT) 168
compassion, self- 97, 102
composting 11–14
concrete spaces 34
Conn, L. 73
Conn, S. 73
connection and belonging, feelings of 56–58, 122; *see also* attachment-informed environmental arts therapy
Connell, C. 29
Connell, T. O. 170
contact styles **129–130**
CORE outcome measures 178
co-therapist, nature as 36, 50, 58
Cox, D. T. C. 151
creative arts therapies 171; with children (*see* children); emergence of environmental arts therapy from 29–31; ethical practice in 38–39; natural materials in 55–56, 57; nature mask 50–51, *51*; risk and benefit assessment of 39–40
culture of narcissism 127–128
cybernetics 206

Davies, J. 9, 30, 32
Dawkins, P. 201
Daytime Community Therapies 13
death: approaching, in elderhood 210–211; leaf of 188–191, *190*, *191*, 193–196, *194*, *195*; by suicide in children 49; threat of 98; turning year cycle and 10, 25; *see also* palliative care
Death Mother 82
decentring 144–145
depression, Mind in the City workshops on 161, 162
'Descent of Inanna' myth 95–96
developmental psychology 49
Devon Partnership Trust 13, 21
disability arts 14
Divine Beauty: The Invisible Embrace 89
Divine feminine 88
Dracula 188
dramatherapy 13–14, 32
"Drawing Nature" 30
Dreamtime Theatre 13–14
drug induced psychosis 21
duty of care 38

Earth as living entity 67, 76, 165
Earth Talks-Indigenous Ways of Knowing, The 88

EarthWays 62; ascent through the woods in 66; body and emotion in 64–65; encounter in 66–68; flow of feeling in 65–66; love, attachment and loss as the field in 62–64; path out of the woods in 71–73; play in 66, 68–70; returning to the field with another perspective in 75–76; ritual and myth in 66, 70–71; seeing the field through new eyes in 73–74, *75*
Easter 15, 158
eco-art therapy 30, 39
Eco-art Therapy: Creativity that let the Earth Teach 30
ecological self 48, 50, 73
ecology 27–28; of imagination 29
Ecominds project 152
ecopsychology 27–28, 169, 170
ecotherapy 9, 27–28, 169–170
Ecotherapy Theory, Research and Practice 74
effigies 18–19
eggs as new beginnings 15–17, 158, 162
Elbrecht, C. 53
elders, reflections on work as 209–211
elder women's group: elder womanhood explored in 200–203, *202*; facilitation of 203; introduction to 197; moving deeper and deeper 203–205, *204*; moving outwards 205–208; reflections on work as elders in 209–211; roots of 197–199; sacred places in 205; story of the wood and 199–200; summary of 211–212; therapeutic potential of trees and 200
Eliade, M. 205
Ellis, C. 107
emerging 14–18
emotional geographies 139
emotions, letting go of suppressed 97–99
empathic identification 73–74, *75*
enactment 111
encounter in EarthWays 66–68
environmental arts therapy: as action-oriented therapy 114; in adult mental health services (*see* mental health services, outdoor art therapy in adult); attachment-informed (*see* attachment-informed environmental arts therapy); Circle of Trees (*see* Circle of Trees groups); defined 1, 33; ecology, ecopsychology and ecotherapies in 27–28; elder women's group (*see* elder women's group); emergence from field of creative arts therapies 29–31; ethical practice in 38–39; framework

of 169–170; health benefits of working in nature and 36–38; as integrative creative arts therapy 2; nature as outside frame in 35–36; nurturing a reciprocal relationship 28–29; our shadow nature and need for 121–122; in palliative care (*see* palliative care); risk and benefit assessment of 39–40, 171; solar and lunar time in 127–128, **129–130**, 131; storytelling in 123–127; trauma-informed (*see* trauma-informed environmental arts therapy); twelve monthly cycles in 131–132; wilderness therapy (*see* wilderness therapy); *see also* art therapy outdoors
"Environmental Arts Therapy, Metaphors in the Field" 9, 30
Environmental Arts Therapy and the Tree of Life 9, 11, 18, 33, 123, 131, 148, 169
Environmental Arts Therapy UK 25
environmental crisis 10, 25, 82
Eostra festival 15
ethical practice 38–39
Exeter Health Authority 13

fantasies 30, 35, 143
fathers *see* wilderness therapy
fatigue, effects of nature on 37
fears 30, 35, 143
felt meaning 171
fertility symbols 158
Five Ways to Wellbeing model 152–153, 160
flowering 18–21
foraging of art materials 155
forest bathing 38
fossil fuels 76
frames, therapeutic 34–35; nature as 'outside' 35–36
Franz, M. L. 48
Friedman, N. 171
fruiting 22–25
Fuller, R. A. 151
functional magnetic resonance imaging (fMRI) 94

Gaia as good enough mother 86–87
Gaston, K. J. 151
gestalt cycle 132, 148
gestalt group therapy 200
Gestalt psychotherapy 121
Gifford, R. 97
Gilbert, P. 97
Gill, T. 39–40

grandmother, concept of 201–202
Graves, R. 17
Greek mythology 159
Greenberg, L. S. 101
Green Studio 32, 140
'green studio' 32
grief ritual 14
Griffiths, J. 73
groupwork, outdoor art therapy 40
Guardian, The 76
Guattari, F. 29

Hackney and Waltham Forest 159–160
Hageneder, F. 34
Hallow'een 23
Hasbach, P. 38, 39, 40
Haugen, M. G. 205
Healing Forest, The 37
healing process of creativity 29
Health and Care Professions Council (HCPC) 38
health benefits of working in nature 36–38
Heart Leaves 174
heart-opening with nature 123
Heritage of Trees, The 34
Hidden Life of Trees, The 67–68
hidden self, searching for the 112–114
Highgate Wood, London 11, 139–140
Hilgers, L. 50
Hillman, J. 49
Hillyer, C. 200
hippocampus 53
Holbeam Woods, Devon 25
Homunculus 20–21
Hougham, R. 108
Hudson, H. L. 151
human-nature relatedness 28; as reciprocal relationship 28–29

identification, empathic 73–74, *75*
imagination, nature inspiring 55
Imbolc festival 14
indigenous art form 9
indigenous cultures 30, 33, 73
inherent selves 123–124
initiation 119
inner child, connecting to 23, 32, 73
inner frame in art therapy 35
inner tyrants 80–83
integrated self 121–122, 132–133
Intergovernmental Panel on Climate Change (IPCC) 76
International Association 33

interoception 98–99, 102
Ispirescu, P. 185

Jacobs, L. 207–208
Jennings, S. 68, 70
Johnson, D. R. 68
Johnstone, C. 206
Jones, P. 110
Jones, V. 31, 40, 140, 170, 198–199
Jordan, M. 28, 36–37, 41, 95, 138–139, 146,
    163–164, 168–169, 180
Jung, C. G. 48, 53, 88, 106, 113–114, 181
Jung, E. 88

Kalmanowitz, D. 35, 113
Kaplan, H. 30
Kaplan, R. 36
Kaplan, S. 36, 170
Kelly, D. 198
Kerényi, C. 71
Kopytin, A. 31, 32, 39, 49

Lahad, M. 37, 41
Lammas festival 22, 34
lay of the land 138–139
leaf mounds 12
leaf of death 188–191, *190*, *191*
Levine, P. A. 94, 98, 99
Li, Q. 38
Licata, M. 82
Lionheart men's group 12
listening 131
Lloyd, B. 35, 113
London Art Therapy Centre 11, 25, 33, 169
Louv, R. 37, 49, 53
lunar and solar time 127–128, **129–130**, 131

Macy, J. 73, 76, 206
magic imp 74, *75*
Marshall, H. 95, 168
Maryon Park community gardens 163–164,
    165
mask, nature 50–51, *51*
Maslow, A. H. 69
Maté, G. 103
McCabe, P. 88–89
McNiff, S. 4–5, 29, 49
meditation, playful absorption as 69
Meetup 164
men, environmental art therapy for 21; *see
    also* wilderness therapy
'me-not me' experiences 57
mental health services, outdoor art
    therapy in adult 37; co-facilitating and

occupational therapy outdoors in 175;
    conclusions on 180–181; development
    of 172–173, 175–178; introduction
    to 167–169, *168*; locations and
    experiences in 173–174; outcomes
    and group processes in 175, 178–180;
    referrals and risk assessment in 173,
    178; transportation and evaluation
    174–175, 178
mentalisation 71–73
meta-awareness 71–73
metaphor 71, 72, 114, 170; mythologies
    and 146–148, *147*; natural 1, 9, 17, 180;
    natural materials and 145–146
midsummer solstice 20
Milner, M. 35
MIND 21
mindful-meditation practice 31
mindfulness 71–73
Mind in the City workshops 159–163
miniatures, use of 117–118
more-than-human nature 48
mother complex 81
Mother Earth 88–89, 201
mothering ourselves 86–87
mothers *see* Bringing the Outside In
motivation, Mind in the City workshops on
    162–163
Mount Gould Hospital 73
mundus imaginalis 210
Murray, C. 17
Murray, L. 17
music therapy, outdoor 31–32
mythology 71; Greek 159; metaphors and
    146–148, *147*; paganism of Celtic 159;
    Welsh 169

narcissism, culture of 127–128
Nash, G. 25, 169
natural materials: foraging of 155;
    metaphors and 145–146
natural metaphors 1, 9, 17, 180
natural spaces, living and working in
    138–139
nature: complex reality of 72–73; as
    co-therapist 36, 50, 58; culture of
    narcissism and 127–128; decentering
    in 144–145; edges of therapeutic
    encounters in 148–149; emotional
    geographies and 139; feeling of
    belonging with return to 122; health
    benefits of working in 36–38; inspiring
    imagination 55; mental health and (*see*
    mental health services, outdoor art

therapy in); as outside frame 35–36; physicality of body and 141–142; playback recordings of 31–32; sacred places in 205; shared experiences of sensory-emotional responses to 57; silence and solace in 143

Nature-based expressive arts therapy 29, 32–33

nature-deficit-disorder 37, 49

nature mask 50–51, *51*

Naturesense 13–14, 21

nature therapy 32

neuro-biological synchronisation 56

neuroimagery 52

New Economics Foundation 153

Nicholls, V. 170

Nicholson, S. 55

No Fear: Growing Up in a Risk Averse Society 39

objective edges or thresholds 35

occupational therapy 175

O'Donohue, J. 89

Office for National Statistics Online 49

'off-site' scavenging 30

O'Flaherty, R. 17

Ogden, P. 98

Ogygia 17

optimal attachment communications 56

Orians, G. 52

Outdoor Music Therapy (OdMT) 31–32

outer frame in art therapy 35; nature as 35–36

paganism 159

pain 83–86; of the wounded feminine 100–101

palliative care: introduction to 185–186; leaf of death and 188–191, *190*, *191*, 193–196, *194*, *195*; staff environmental arts therapy workshop for 191–193; Tree of Life model and 186–188

Park, B. J. 38

Pearson, J. 107

Perera, S. B. 99–100

Pfeifer, E. 31–32, 36

physical illness *see* trauma-informed environmental arts therapy

physicality of body and earth 141–142

Pinkola Estes, C. 81, 87, 201

playback recordings 31–32

play in EarthWays 66, 68–70

Pope, A. 200

portable studios 35

Potter, T. 170

Prentice, H. 73

projections 30, 35, 143

projective work 70, 98

psychic space 50

psychobiological states 52

psychodynamic frames 35

psychological hygiene 110

psychotherapy: in elder women's group 206, 209, 211–212; felt meaning in 171; Gestalt 121

public domain, artworks in the 39

putting down roots 83

Queens Wood, London 140

reciprocal relationship, human-nature 4–5, 28–29, 30, 33, 74, 152, 198, 210

reciprocity as elders 210

red tent movement 200

reed boats 24, *24*

reflection 71–73

reptilian brain 52

response-art 148

restorative therapy 170

Resurgence magazine 25, 148

retroflecting 121

risk and benefit assessment 39–40, 171, 173, 178

rites of passage 116

ritual and myth: in attachment-informed environmental arts therapy 66, 70–71; grief 14; in trauma-informed environmental arts therapy 98–100; in wilderness therapy 108

role clarity 110

role-play 97

Roszak, T. 2, 27–28, 50, 67, 73

Rothschild, B. 53

Rugh, M. 31, 32, 49

Russell Clinic 21

Rust, M. J. 28, 148–149

sacred places 205

Sacred Unity, A 206

safety, client 39

Samhain festival 23, 34

Scannell, L. 97

scapegoat 57, 95

'scavenger hunts' 30

Schaverien, J. 35

schizophrenia 21

Schore, A. N. 56

Schroeder, H. W. 167

Scull, J. 72–73
Seager, J. 67
seasonal cycle 41
seasons: attunement to 142; elder women's group and 201–202; moving art therapy outdoors and 142–145, *144*; in twelve monthly cycle 131–132; working with natural cycles of 145–146
secondary intersubjectivity 57
seed gathering and planting 11
self: ecological 48, 50, 73; expansion of 73–74, *75*; going in search of the hidden 112–114; the inherent 123–124; integrated 121–122, 132–133; shadow 179
self-care 97, 102, 186, 193
self-compassion 97, 102
self-deception 148
self-determination 121
self-Nature split 48
self-regulation 206
senses, dull-down 53–54
sensory exercise 31
separation distress 63
shadow self 179
shame 20–21
Shanahan, D. F. 151
Shaw, R. 108
Shepard, P. 57
Shinrin-yoku 38
Siddons Heginworth, I. 11, 33, 214–216; adult mental health services and 168–169; childhood and reflecting upon mother and 88; Circle of Trees and 140, 145–146, 148; elder women's group and 198; integrated self and 123; wounded feminine and 95
silence in nature 143
smell, sense of 38
Snyder, M. 29, 33, 40
social isolation, Mind in the City workshops on 161
solace in nature 143
solar and lunar time 127–128, **129–130**, 131
solstice, midsummer 20
'space between' 108
spatial concepts 35
spears *16*
species extinction 76
Spirit of Trees, The 34
spring equinox 158
Springfield Park, London 154, 158, 160–161, 163

Spring season 142; Mind in the City workshops 160, 162–163
staff environmental arts therapy in palliative care 191–193
storytelling 123–124; purposes of 127; Tapping on the Window 124–126
stress: effects of healthy touch on 53; effects of nature on 37; Mind in the City workshops on 162
Studio Upstairs 153–154, 159
suicide 49
Summer season 142; Maryon Park community gardens and 163–164, *165*
sumpatheia ton hollon 210
Sweeney, T. 30–31, 40, 169, 179
symbols 29–30, 72, 110–111, 114; eggs 15–17, 158, 162; fertility 158

Tapping on the Window 124–126
terminal illness 29, 189, 191
therapeutic frames and boundaries 34–35
third space 36
Thunberg, G. 67
time, solar and lunar 127–128, **129–130**, 131
Totton, N. 34–35, 140
touch: healthy 53; in nature therapy 32; physicality of body and earth and 141–142
'touching nature' 32
traditional festivals 9
Transylvania 185–186; *see also* palliative care
trauma 53, 108–109, 113; *see also* Tree of Life model
trauma-informed environmental arts therapy: ascent in 101–102; case study inquiry into 94; conclusions on 102–104; descending to the underworld in 97–99; encountering the wounded feminine in 100–101; introduction to 93–94; meat hook in 99–100; resourcing for, as suggested by both new and ancient literature 96–97; therapeutic landscape and 95–96
Tree of Life model 186–188; leaf of death and 188–191, *190*, *191*
trees: Celtic Ogham tree calendar 17–18, 34; COATS (Community Outdoor Art Therapy Service) and (*see* COATS (Community Outdoor Art Therapy Service)); in EarthWays (*see* EarthWays); elder women's group and (*see* elder women's group); only knowing the wound and 84–85; symbolism of 29–30; therapeutic potential of 200; Tree of Life model (*see* Tree of Life model); trust and

putting down roots and 83, *84*; as wombs 14–15; *see also* Circle of Trees groups; wilderness therapy

Trevarthen, C. 57

trust 83

Turner, T.-P. 84

turning year cycle outdoor art therapy 33–34, 123–124; composting in 11–14; emerging in 14–18; flowering in 18–21; fruiting in 22–25, *24*; introduction to 9–11; *see also* seasons

twelve monthly cycles *see* seasons

urban spaces 139–141, 151–152; Studio Upstairs and 153–154; *see also* COATS (Community Outdoor Art Therapy Service)

Val Huet 191–192

Van der Kolk, B. 72, 94, 96, 97

Ventura, M. 49

Verhaagen, D. 110

vernal equinox 158

walking: aware 31; effects of, on fatigue and stress 37

wall, the 22–23

war, effects of 32

Warwick Edinburgh Mental Wellbeing Scale (WEMWEBS) 178

Welsh mythology 169

Whitaker, P. 39

White Goddess, The 17

wild Amazonian man 54–55

wilderness therapy 170; breaking through the barrier 114–116; conclusions on 119; entering the theatre of the wilderness in 107–108; finding the man you want to be through 111–112; finding your father's shadow through 116–118; going in search of your hidden self in 112–114; introduction to 106–107; love between father and child explored in 108–111

Wild Things In The Community 21, 25

Wild Things project 21

'Wild Woman' 87

Winnicott, D. W. 63, 171

Winter season 142

Wohlleben, P. 67–68, 70

womanhood 200–203

womb, tree as 14–15

Women Who Run with The Wolves 81

Wonford House Hospital 21

Woodman, M. 201

Woolley, G. 96

wound, only knowing the 83–86

wounded feminine, the 100–101

Yalom, I. 170, 172

Youth without Age and Life without Death 185, 188